Transplant Care Series

T0122777

Manual of Kidney Transplant Medical Care

Transplant Services, a Unique Partnership of
University of Minnesota Physicians Transplant Program
and Fairview Health Services

Editor: Arthur Matas, MD

Series Editor: Marshall I. Hertz, MD

Science Editor: Laura J. Blakemore, MD

Fairview Publications • *Minneapolis*

Published by Fairview Publications, 2450 Riverside Avenue, Minneapolis, Minnesota 55454. Fairview Publications is a division of Fairview Health Services, a community-focused health system providing a complete range of services, from the prevention of illness and injury to care for the most complex medical conditions.

Library of Congress Cataloging-in-Publication Data
Manual of kidney transplant medical care / Transplant Services, a
  unique partnership of University of Minnesota Physicians
  Transplant Program and Fairview Health Services ; editor,
  Arthur Matas
      p. ; cm. -- (Transplant care series)
  Includes bibliographic references and index.
  ISBN 1-57749-143-2 (spiral bound : alk. paper)
  1. Kidneys--Transplantation--Patients--Medical care--Handbooks,
  manuals, etc.   I. Matas, Arthur, 1948-   . II. University of
  Minnesota Physicians Transplant Program. III. Fairview
  Health Services. IV. Series.
  [DNLM: 1. Kidney Transplantation--methods--Handbooks. 2.
Immunosuppression--methods--Handbooks. 3. Postoperative
Care--methods--Handbooks. 4. Preoperative Care--methods--
Handbooks.   WJ 39 M2939 2003]
  RD575.M35 2003
  617.4'610592--dc21

2003010327

First Printing: October 2003
Printed in the United States of America
07 06 05 04 03   6 5 4 3 2 1

Cover by Laurie Ingram Design, www.laurieingramdesign.com
Typeset by Corey Sevett, Artisan Creative Computer Services

For a free current catalog of Fairview Publications titles, please call toll-free
1-800-544-8207. Or visit our Web site at www.fairviewpress.org.

Funding for this book provided by the Academic Health Center of the University of Minnesota and Fairview Health Services.

The authors acknowledge the contributions of the following professionals who participated in the development of this manual:

Blanche Chavers, MD
Marie Cook, RN, CPNP, MPH, CCTC
Catherine Garvey, RN, BA, CCTC
Abhinav Humar, MD
Cheryl Jacobs, MSW, LICSW
Raja Kandaswamy, MD
Bert Kasiske, MD
Melissa Kennedy, PharmD, BCPS
Rahul Koushik, MD
Heather Mittica, MSW

Medical Disclaimer

Medscape

Fairview Publications is a member of the Medscape Publishers' Circle, an alliance of leading medical publishers whose content is featured on Medscape (http://www.medscape.com). Medscape is part of the WebMD Medscape Health Network, the leading online healthcare resource for professionals and consumers.

Contents

Introduction

Kidney transplantation is the treatment of choice for patients with end-stage kidney disease. Compared to dialysis, transplantation provides increased longevity and a markedly better quality of life. More transplant (vs. dialysis) patients are able to return to an active lifestyle in their community, school, or the workforce. In some situations, the improvement in survival with transplantation vs. dialysis is dramatic (e.g., patients with diabetes). In others, there are specific reasons why transplantation is preferred (e.g., improved growth in children).

The first successful transplant was done between identical twins in 1954. It was almost a decade later before development of immunosuppressive protocols allowed non-twin transplants. Since then, there has been incremental improvement in both patient and graft survival with the use of new immunosuppressive agents, the introduction of better protocols (and agents) for infection prophylaxis, and the development of improved patient care algorithms. Currently, 1-year patient and graft survival rates are more than 90%.

The purpose of this manual is to provide basic information regarding the care of kidney transplant recipients at the University of Minnesota/Fairview-University Medical Center Transplant Program. Our goal is to highlight the algorithms we use in donor and recipient evaluation and in the postoperative care of the kidney transplant recipient.

The manual provides information about how to contact our program for both pre- and posttransplant issues. It describes the pretransplant evaluation of adult and pediatric recipients, the evaluation and care of kidney donors, our current immunosuppressive protocols and the individual drugs used, and the long-term care and outcomes of kidney transplant recipients.

A large part of our program has always been research to improve outcomes for kidney transplant recipients. Consequently, our protocols are constantly evolving. We plan to revise and update this manual regularly to reflect these changes. Please send comments, suggestions, and other correspondence to:

Arthur J. Matas, MD
Department of Surgery
University of Minnesota/Fairview-University Medical Center
11-200 Phillips-Wangensteen Building, MMC 328
420 Delaware Street SE
Minneapolis, MN 55455
Phone 612.625.6460
Fax 612.624.7168
Email matas001@umn.edu

I. Program Description

A. Program History

The first kidney transplant at the University of Minnesota/Fairview-University Medical Center (F-UMC), formerly the University of Minnesota Hospital and Clinics, was performed in 1963. Since then, we have done more than 6000 transplants including more than 3000 transplants from living donors.[1,2] The program is one of the oldest and largest in the world.

Since its inception, a major goal of the program has been to improve short- and long-term outcomes for transplant recipients. We have pioneered kidney transplantation for infants and children, high-risk recipients, and patients with diabetes. We have studied new immunosuppressive and infection prophylaxis agents as they became available and then introduced them into our clinical trials. And we have maintained our extensive clinical database of both retrospective and prospective studies, which is designed to improve recipient outcomes. Consequently, our program has seen incremental improvement in patient and graft survival, with simultaneous decreases in morbidity. We continue to maintain a commitment to research to improve outcomes for future patients.

B. The Transplant Center

B.1. Function

The Transplant Center coordinates the care of kidney transplant recipients. This includes maintaining regular contact with referring and primary care physicians, who participate in the pre- and posttransplant care of transplant recipients.

B.2. Contact information

For general information, new referrals, questions regarding patients awaiting a transplant, or follow-up information about transplant recipients, contact the Transplant Center at the following address or telephone numbers:

Kidney Transplant Program
Transplant Center
University of Minnesota/Fairview-University Medical Center
Mayo Mail Code 482
420 Delaware Street SE
Minneapolis, MN 55455

Local phone	612.625.5115
Toll-free phone	1.800.328.5465
Office hours:	Monday through Friday, 8:00 A.M. to 4:30 P.M. (Central Time)

B.3 Kidney transplant team

A multidisciplinary approach ensures optimal patient care. The members of the kidney transplant team and their phone numbers are as follows:

Transplant Surgeons

David L. Dunn, MD, PhD	612.626.1999
Rainer W. Gruessner, MD	612.625.1485
Abhinav Humar, MD	612.624.0688
Raja Kandaswamy, MD	612.625.7997
Arthur J. Matas, MD	612.625.6460
John S. Najarian, MD, PhD	612.625.8444
William D. Payne, MD	612.625.5151
David Sutherland, MD, PhD	612.625.7600

Adult Nephrologists

Hassan Ibrahim, MD	612.624.9444
Bert Kasiske, MD	612.624.9444
Rahul Koushik, MD	612.624.9444
Connie Manske, MD	612.624.9444
Mark Rosenberg, MD	612.624.9444

Pediatric Nephrologists

Michael Bendel-Stenzel, MD	612.626.2922
Blanche Chavers, MD	612.626.2922
Elizabeth Ingulli, MD	612.626.2922
Clifford Kashtan, MD	612.626.2922
Michael Mauer, MD	612.626.2922
Thomas Nevins, MD	612.626.2922

Adult Transplant Coordinators

Louise Berry, RN	612.625.5115
Mary Beth Drangstveit, RN, CCTC	612.625.5115
Catherine Garvey, RN, CCTC	612.625.5115
Pandora Halverson, RN	612.625.5115
Maureen Hayes, RN	612.625.5115
Mary Huepfel, RN	612.625.5115
Marilyn Leister, RN	612.625.5115
Erin Norris, RN	612.625.5115
Sarah Peterson, LPN	612.625.5115
Mary Rolf, RN, CCTC	612.625.5115
Marci Siers, RN	612.625.5115
Dawn Thell, RN	612.625.5115

Pediatric Transplant Coordinators

Marie Cook, RN, CPNP, MPH, CCTC	612.625.4166
Marci Knaak, RN	612.625.8666

Social Workers

Angela Herr, MSW	612.273.3366
Cheryl Jacobs, MSW, LICSW	612.273.5325
Ed Maxwell, MSW, LICSW	612.273.3366
Kathy Weck, MSW	612.273.4936

B.4 Organ donation information

LifeSource, our regional organ-procurement organization, makes the match between donor organs and individuals awaiting transplant. LifeSource is responsible for managing all organ donation activities in Minnesota, North Dakota, and South Dakota.

If transplant recipients would like to send an anonymous thank-you to their donor family, a brochure entitled "Writing to Donor Families" is available from their transplant coordinator or directly from LifeSource. This brochure offers advice on writing to donor families and provides information about how to send such correspondence.

For more information about the donation process and how you can help educate the public about organ donation, contact LifeSource at the following address or telephone numbers:

> LifeSource
> 2550 University Avenue West
> Suite 315 South
> St. Paul, MN 55114-1904
> 651.603.7800 or 1.800.24SHARE

ARTHUR MATAS, MD

References

1. Moss A, Najarian JS, Sutherland DER, Payne WD, Gruessner RWG, Humar A, Kandaswamy R, Gillingham KJ, Dunn DL, Matas AJ. 5,000 kidney transplants—a single-center experience. In: Cecka and Terasaki, eds. *Clinical Transplants 2000.* Los Angeles, CA: UCLA Immunogenetics Center; 2001.

2. Matas AJ, Payne WD, Sutherland DER, Humar A, Gruessner RWG, Kandaswamy R, Dunn DL, Gillingham KJ, Najarian JS. 2,500 living donor kidney transplants—a single-center experience. *Ann Surg.* 2001;234(2):149-164.

II. Pretransplant Issues

The goal of the pretransplant evaluation is to optimize the patient's overall medical status and anticipate problems that could be addressed between the time of the pretransplant evaluation and the actual transplantation. Some of these medical problems may not be related to the kidneys but may affect the patient's postoperative course. In general, these guidelines and policies are in accordance with the recently published "Evaluation of Renal Transplant Candidates: Clinical Practice Guidelines," which have been endorsed by the American Society of Transplantation.[1]

A. When to Refer

It is now clear that, in both adults and children, outcomes after preemptive transplantation are better than outcomes after transplantation preceded by dialysis.[2] But perfectly timed cadaveric transplantation is often not possible due to the long waiting times required to receive a cadaveric kidney. Therefore, it is reasonable to begin the planning of renal replacement therapy (RRT) at an early stage. The current guideline is to refer these patients for RRT 6 to 12 months before the need for renal replacement is anticipated. This roughly corresponds to a glomerular filtration rate (GFR) of 30 mL per minute or chronic kidney disease Stage 4 based on the National Kidney Foundation's classification system.[3]

To accrue time on the United Network for Organ Sharing (UNOS) waiting list, patients must have an estimated or measured GFR that is not more than 20 mL per minute. However, it may be prudent to get added to the waiting list earlier on the outside chance of receiving a 6-antigen matched kidney. The current National Kidney Foundation guidelines recommend using the serum creatinine (Cr) concentration to calculate the GFR based on age, gender, race, and/or body weight.[3] A formula such as the Cockcroft-Gault[4] formula (1) or the Modification of Diet in Renal Disease (MDRD)[5] formula (2) may be used to estimate an adult's GFR as follows:

(1) GFR = 0.84 x [Cockcroft-Gault C_{Cr} (mL/min) = (140-age) x body weight/(72 x Cr), multiplied by 0.85 if female, where age is in years, body weight is in kilograms, and serum creatinine (Cr) is in mg/dL]

(2) MDRD GFR = 170 x $[P_{Cr}]^{-0.999}$ x $[Age]^{-0.176}$ x [0.762 if patient is female] x [1.180 if patient is black] x $[SUN]^{-0.17}$ x $[Alb]^{+0.318}$

Calculators for determining the GFR are located at http://nephron.com/mdrd/default.html.

Under special conditions such as oxalosis, patients may be referred at an earlier stage to derive maximum benefit from transplantation.

B. Criteria for Referral

B.1. Age

Children older than 5 years have undergone successful transplantation. At present, there is no upper age limit for kidney transplantation at the University of Minnesota/Fairview-University Medical Center. Older patients usually undergo a more extensive cardiac evaluation and more frequent review while on the waiting list.

B.2. Cancer

Immunosuppression increases morbidity and mortality associated with cancer. For most potentially life-threatening cancers, an appropriate disease-free interval of 2 years after a documented cure is reasonable to reduce this risk. In patients with certain cancers, such as breast, invasive cervical, or colorectal cancer, a 5-year waiting period may be necessary. Patients with basal cell carcinomas or incidentally discovered renal cell cancers smaller than 5 cm do not need to undergo a waiting period.

B.3. Primary kidney disease

Although a number of primary kidney diseases have high recurrence rates in the allograft, most recurrences do not cause graft failure. A notable exception is focal segmental glomerulosclerosis (FSGS), which has a recurrence rate of 20% to 40% and poses a 40% to 50% risk of graft loss.[6] There is some evidence that early treatment with plasma exchange may reduce the rate of allograft loss. At present, we do not consider FSGS to be a contraindication to transplantation. A possible exception is FSGS that has already caused allograft failure. In these instances, the chance of recurrence is at least 75%, making careful evaluation of the risks and benefits of a second transplantation necessary.

Hemolytic uremic syndrome (HUS), despite a high recurrence rate and a 50% rate of graft failure, is not considered a contraindication to transplantation. Primary oxalosis is cured with combined liver-kidney transplantation, if there is renal insufficiency, and isolated liver transplantation, if renal function is normal. We currently recommend early referral of these patients for transplant evaluation, when MDRD GFR is <50 mL/min.

B.4. Viral illnesses

Hepatitis B and C generally do not preclude transplantation. However, these patients need careful evaluation, and a liver biopsy is often indicated to assess the risk of immunosuppressive therapy. Some patients may require disease-modulating therapies concurrent or prior to transplantation. Such therapy is best planned with advanced referral and can be coordinated in conjunction with a hepatologist. Human immunodeficiency virus (HIV)-positive patients with a controlled viral load are sometimes candidates for kidney transplantation.

B.5. Coronary artery disease

Coronary artery disease is the leading cause of death after renal transplantation. Available data suggest that revascularization prior to transplantation may reduce the risk of posttransplant coronary heart disease events. Therefore, it has been our policy that patients with critical coronary lesions undergo revascularization prior to transplantation. A cardiologist evaluates all patients referred for transplantation. Low-risk patients are generally screened via a noninvasive cardiac stress test. High-risk patients may be asked to undergo coronary angiography, with or without stress testing.

B.6. Other considerations

With the shortage of organ donors and the long waiting times for cadaveric kidneys, transplantation across cross-match and blood group barriers may be considered. Protocols for improving graft survival in recipients who have exhausted all other sources of potential donors are currently underway.

C. Pretransplant Medical Evaluation

A detailed medical evaluation is carried out prior to deciding whether the patient is a suitable candidate for transplantation. If desired, a significant portion of the evaluation can be performed at the referring medical facility. Tests and consultations that are generally done at Fairview-University Medical Center are marked with an asterisk.

C.1. Consultations*

- Kidney transplant surgeon.
- Transplant nephrologist.
- Transplant coordinator.
- Kidney transplant social worker.
- Financial representative.

Consultation with other health care professionals, if required, can be easily arranged. All patients see a cardiologist.

C.2. Laboratory tests

The following laboratory tests are part of a standard pretransplant evaluation:

- Complete blood count (CBC).
- Chemistry profile including electrolytes, blood urea nitrogen (BUN), and creatinine (Cr).
- Complete liver function tests including liver enzymes, bilirubin, albumin, and international normalized ratio (INR).
- Coagulation profile including partial thromboplastin time (PTT) and fibrinogen levels.
- Blood group typing and cross matching.
- Viral serology for hepatitis A, B, and C; cytomegalovirus (CMV); Epstein-Barr virus (EBV); and human immunodeficiency virus (HIV).
- Glycosylated hemoglobin for diabetic patients.
- Prostate-specific antigen (PSA) for men 55 years or older and those with risk factors.
- Serum pregnancy test for all adolescent girls and women younger than 55 years.
- Fasting lipid profile.
- Uric acid, amylase, lipase, phosphorus, and magnesium levels.
- Panel reactive antibody.*
- Human leukocyte antigen (HLA) typing.*

C.3. Imaging studies and other procedures

- Chest radiograph (x-ray).
- Pulmonary function tests (for smokers or people with pulmonary problems).
- Electrocardiogram (ECG).
- Coronary angiogram (if indicated by cardiac consult, if a diabetic older than 45 years, or if a diabetic with a 25 pack-year smoking history).
- Abdominal ultrasound.
- Femoral Doppler study (if a history of peripheral vascular disease).
- Voiding cystourethrogram (VCUG; if a history of recurrent infections, reflux, or congenital abnormalities).
- Pelvic examination or Pap smear (if not done within past year).
- Mammogram in all women older than 40 years.

C.4. Other tests

- Urinalysis.
- Urine culture.
- Stool guaiac test (x 3).
- Glomerular filtration rate (GFR) calculation.
- Purified protein derivative (PPD) skin test with controls for mumps and *Candida*.

C.5. Vaccinations

- Hepatitis B vaccine (Recombivax Hb), if never vaccinated or hepatitis B surface antigen (HbsAg)-negative.
- Pneumococcal vaccine (Pneumovax), if not already vaccinated within past 5 to 10 years.

D. The Role of the Primary Physician

D.1. Prepare for referral

We believe that the primary physician or nephrologist plays a critical role in the pretransplant evaluation. An initial information session to briefly discuss the options available—namely, dialysis and transplantation—with their risks and benefits, should be made available as soon as it has been determined that the patient's likelihood of needing renal replacement therapy is very high. At this time, important barriers, such as ischemic heart disease (critical), substance abuse, medication noncompliance, and behavioral issues, should be identified and controlled. Once these issues are stabilized, the patient can be referred for a pretransplant evaluation.

D.2. Review options and risks

A common area in which we encourage all of the involved health personnel to take a proactive role is counseling the patient about weight loss and smoking cessation. Both obesity and cigarette smoking have been identified as modifiable risk factors for poor outcomes after transplantation.

It is also important for the primary physician to make the potential recipient aware of the shortage of cadaveric kidneys and the need to consider living-donor transplantation whenever possible. It is now clear that emotionally related kidney donation by a spouse or a close friend is as beneficial as a living-related kidney donation in terms of long-term survival. With the use of laparoscopic donor surgery, which is now routinely performed at the University of Minnesota/Fairview-University

Medical Center, donor morbidity has been reduced. Moreover, the waiting time on the transplant list is likely to lengthen with the diminishing pool of available kidneys. The current wait time for a cadaveric kidney ranges from 3 to 5 years.

E. Pretransplant Psychosocial Evaluation

All potential transplant recipients undergo a psychosocial assessment by a clinical social worker at the initial transplant work-up. This assessment includes examination of the recipient's current life situation and motivation for seeking a transplant. In addition, the patient's psychological, familial, social, and employment history are reviewed. The importance of having family and social support available is emphasized, while available transplant resources are also made known to the patient and family.

Transplantation can place a financial burden on a patient and family. The individual's financial situation, including medication coverage and health insurance, is also carefully reviewed during the evaluation. Financial issues can arise from lost wages (due to time away from work) and the expense of life-long immunosuppressive therapy, so it is crucial that the potential candidate have a thorough understanding of the financial implications of transplantation. Employment, rehabilitation, and insurance issues are also discussed with prospective recipients.

The clinician may identify potential factors that identify a candidate at risk for graft rejection (e.g., history of noncompliance with treatment, inadequate resources or social support). Some patients may warrant further intervention prior to becoming a transplant candidate and may be referred for appropriate treatment (i.e., psychological support, chemical dependency rehabilitation). The patient should be able to demonstrate adherence to their medical regimen of clinic visits, dialysis, fluid/diet restrictions, and medication administration when determining transplant candidacy.

Any recommendations are made known to the patient and the treating physician. This is to ensure that patients understand what is expected of them before they become transplant candidates.

F. Psychosocial Assistance and Patient Resources

Given the significant impact of kidney transplantation on the lives of the recipients and their families, a variety of types of psychosocial support and assistance is offered.

F.1. Discharge planning and social services

Social work services and discharge planning assistance are available to all kidney transplant recipients while hospitalized. Discharge planning includes linkage to community resources, or assistance with placement in a transitional or long-term care facility when necessary. RN care coordinators are also available to arrange home care and follow-up appointments after discharge.

Posttransplant, there may be ongoing issues related to adjustment to illness, re-entry into the work force, change in life roles, and financial concerns. Social workers can provide supportive and interventional services to posttransplant recipients, as well as link them to community resources. Patients should be encouraged to contact their transplant social worker if they experience any psychosocial concerns. Counseling to help patients adjust to transplantation is made available.

F.2. Financial issues

All transplant recipients are assigned a patient financial representative (PFR) who assists them with obtaining insurance approval for their transplant. The PFR is also available to recipients during their first posttransplant year. Most kidney transplant recipients are eligible for Medicare End-Stage Renal Disease (ESRD) benefits. The PFR or social worker can instruct the patient on how to apply for Medicare and explain coverage benefits.

Some recipients may be eligible for other financial assistance or transplant grants to help with their particular circumstance. They should contact their social worker to learn if they qualify for additional financial help.

Patients should contact their transplant social worker as soon as they identify any insurance or medication coverage concerns. It is important that he or she assist them in obtaining appropriate resources *before* they no longer have adequate coverage or recourses. Some patients become at great risk for losing their graft because they can no longer pay for their immunosuppressive medications.

F.3. Outpatient Specialty Pharmacy/medications

Fairview-University Medical Center (F-UMC) has a Specialty Pharmacy service tailored to the needs of transplant patients. Patients are dispensed a 1-month supply of medications at discharge; subsequent medications are shipped to the patient's home at no cost. The Specialty Pharmacy is able to accept most insurance plans, including out-of-state providers.

As the recipient nears discharge from the hospital, a pharmacist meets with the transplant recipient to discuss the Specialty Pharmacy program and offer the patient the option to enroll in it. (There is no charge for this service.) Enrolled patients are provided a toll-free number they can call to speak with a pharmacist at any time: 612.626.2177 or 1.888.783.2974.

After discharge, a program pharmacist contacts the patient a week before the first refill is needed to review medications with the patient, monitor for compliance, and reorder required medications. Specialty pharmacists also work closely with transplant coordinators and social workers to coordinate care and resolve any problems. This monthly monitoring is provided on an ongoing basis.

Patients enrolled in the Specialty Pharmacy program are also assigned a patient financial advocate (PFA) and a transplant insurance billing specialist, who are available to answer questions about insurance coverage and complete insurance paperwork. Pharmacy representatives are also available to assist patients with limited financial resources to obtain coverage for their medications.

Transplant recipients who have Medicare Part B will have 80% coverage of only their immunosuppressive medications. (Patients should discuss these types of restrictions with their pharmaceutical representative or social worker.) Some pharmaceutical companies offer indigent medication assistance programs for qualifying individuals.

F.4. Accommodations

Fairview-University Medical Center has an accommodations department that individuals are encouraged to contact if they or their significant others need assistance with lodging during their hospital visit. Many of the hotels in proximity to the hospital provide shuttle service. For assistance, contact: 1.800.328.5576 or 612.273.3695.

Patients who have state Medical Assistance (or Medicaid) may be eligible for county assistance or reimbursement for lodging, travel, and meals; they should discuss this with their county caseworker. Patients should also inform their transplant social worker if they require financial assistance while receiving care at the hospital.

G. Periodic Reevaluation While on the Transplant Waiting List

G.1. When to contact the transplant coordinator

Because patients on the transplant waiting list often remain on dialysis for a long time, they frequently experience dialysis-related complications. Those on peritoneal dialysis may develop peritonitis and those on hemodialysis, access infections. The transplant coordinator should be informed any time a patient is hospitalized, develops an infection, experiences worsening of their medical condition, or has a change in insurance coverage. All of these situations could call for reevaluation of the patient's medical condition prior to transplantation. Such communication helps to optimize the patient's status and avoids disappointment due to last-minute cancellations of surgery due to medical reasons.

G.2. Cardiac monitoring

Patients with coronary artery disease (CAD), as well as those at high risk for developing it, frequently require periodic noninvasive cardiac stress testing.[7] Although this is usually determined at the time of the initial evaluation, we also rely on the patient's primary care physician to contact the transplant coordinator if new cardiac complications develop.

RAHUL KOUSHIK, MD; CATHERINE GARVEY, RN, BA, CCTC;
HEATHER MITTICA, MSW; AND BERT KASISKE, MD

References:

1. Kasiske BL, Cangro CB, Hariharan S, et al. Evaluation of renal transplant candidates: clinical practice guidelines. *Am J Transplant.* 2001;1(s2):5-95.

2. Kasiske BL, Snyder J, Matas AJ, et al. Preemptive kidney transplantation: the advantage and the advantaged. *J Am Soc Nephrol.* 2002;13:1358-64.

3. NKF-K/DOQI (National Kidney Foundation-Kidney Disease Outcomes Quality Initiative) Chronic Kidney Disease Work Group. K/DOQI clinical practice guidelines for chronic kidney disease: evaluation, classification, and stratification. Kidney Disease Outcome Quality Initiative. *Am J Kidney Dis.* 2002 Feb;39(2 suppl 1):S1-246.

4. Cockcroft DW, Gault MH. Prediction of creatinine clearance from serum creatinine. *Nephron.* 1976;16:31-41.

5. Levey AS, Bosch JP, Lewis JB, Greene T, Rogers N, Roth D. A more accurate method to estimate glomerular filtration rate from serum creatinine: a new prediction equation. *Ann Intern Med.* 1999;130(6):461-470.

6. Briganti EM, Russ GR, McNeil JJ, et al. Risk of renal allograft loss from recurrent glomerulonephritis. *N Engl J Med.* 2002;347(2):103-109.

7. Herzog CA, Marwick TH, Pheley AM, et al. Dobutamine stress echocardiography for the detection of significant coronary artery disease in renal transplant candidates. *Am J Kidney Dis.* 1999;33(6):1080-1090.

III. Kidney Donor Evaluation

A. Who Are Donor Candidates?

Any healthy person is a potential kidney donor, including relatives, coworkers, friends, and acquaintances. Our institution also has a program (i.e., Nondirected Donor Program) that accepts individuals who wish to anonymously donate to our cadaveric waiting list. The type of relationship or circumstance will be examined during the donor's medical and psychosocial evaluation.

Volunteers interested in donating a kidney begin the evaluation process when they contact the Transplant Center. (Upon referral, recipients are instructed to have any potential donors contact the Transplant Center for information, as the decision to donate an organ must be voluntary on the part of the donor.) A donor team not involved in the recipient's care subsequently evaluates the potential donor's candidacy and related health issues. Upon completion of this evaluation, the donor team reviews the results and then approves or denies the request to donate a kidney. If a clinical problem was identified during the course of the donor evaluation, the donor is referred to the appropriate care.

B. Donor Screening/Contraindications

Potential donors are screened by the Transplant Center for obvious contraindications to proceeding with transplantation, such as:

- High blood pressure/hypertension.
- Human immunodeficiency virus (HIV) infection or a history of HIV high risk-related behaviors.
- Known viral infections (e.g., hepatitis B or C, Lyme disease).
- Active alcohol or substance abuse.
- Psychiatric illness, psychosocial situation, or impaired mental status that may influence judgment or compromise recovery.
- History of malignancy/cancer (exception: skin cancer).
- Heart or lung disease requiring medications.
- Diabetes mellitus.
- Inappropriate motivation for donation.

Donors also receive educational materials that review the evaluation process and financial issues related to kidney donation, as well as the potential benefits and surgical risks to the donor and recipient. A list of donors is available for potential donors who wish to learn more about donation first-hand.

C. Donor Evaluation

C.1. Donor blood testing

The evaluation of a donor begins with blood testing to assess for compatibility. Blood type is determined, and the donor and recipient are cross-matched. Despite new and emerging protocols to allow transplant using blood type-incompatible donors (or despite positive cross-matches), a compatible donor is always preferred.

C.2. Medical evaluation of donor

The medical evaluation of the donor can be performed where the donor lives, although it is preferably conducted at the Transplant Center. The evaluation includes a thorough medical history and physical examination, extensive laboratory work, urine testing, and radiological examinations, as well as consultations with specialists.

The tests included in the evaluation are:

- Complete metabolic panel including electrolytes, blood urea nitrogen (BUN), and creatinine (Cr).
- Hemogram and platelet count.
- Liver function tests and uric acid.
- Fasting lipid levels.
- International normalized ratio (INR) and partial thromboplastin time (PTT).
- Viral serology for hepatitis B and C, and human immuno-deficiency virus (HIV).
- Rapid plasma reagin (RPR) test.
- Urinalysis.
- Clean-catch urine culture.
- Prostate-specific antigen (PSA) level (for all men >55 years).
- Serum pregnancy test (for all adolescent girls and women ≤55 years).
- Electrocardiogram (ECG).
- Chest radiograph (posteroanterior [PA] and lateral).
- Computed tomography (CT) angiogram and urography.

Donors are screened for diabetes using current American Diabetes Association (ADA) guidelines. In addition, the results of routine cancer surveillance examinations (e.g., mammograms, Pap smears) are requested.

Although any specialist may be consulted during the donor evaluation, most donors see the following individuals:

- Transplant nephrologist.
- Transplant surgeon.
- Transplant coordinator.

- Donor social worker.
- Psychologist.

The potential donors incur no medical expenses, as the Transplant Center covers the cost of the evaluation. In addition, donors are reassured that they can change their mind about being a donor at any time during the evaluation process.

C.3. Psychosocial evaluation of donor

A clinical social worker (not involved in the recipient's care) will conduct a confidential interview to assess the potential donor's motivation, psychological status, and current life situation as it relates to donation. This assessment allows the donor team to better understand individual circumstances that may influence the volunteer's decision to donate. Donation must be entirely voluntary, without pressure from outside sources. To assure informed consent, donors must comprehend information and demonstrate understanding of the risks and potential complications (to donors and recipients) of the procedure. They also must demonstrate the ability to realistically plan for both the surgery and recovery.

During the social work assessment, employment, financial ramifications, family circumstances, available support, and resources are also discussed. If a donor is undergoing psychological treatment (i.e., medication, and/or therapy), the treating mental health professional or physician may be consulted. Each donor's situation is carefully examined. A history of mental health intervention does not necessarily rule out donation, but it may indicate the need for further attention or treatment. If concerns exist, some donors will be asked to see our psychologist to further evaluate their mental status, judgment, and competency.

D. Donor Psychosocial Support

D.1. Inpatient assistance

The donor is admitted to the hospital on the day of surgery and generally stays for 2 to 3 days. Psychosocial services and counseling are available to donors during their hospitalization. There is no need for home care services upon discharge, as the donor is usually capable of managing his or her own postoperative care. However, donors are advised to have a caregiver available for some personal care and driving needs during their recovery due to driving and lifting restrictions. Upon discharge, donors are instructed to not drive for 2 weeks or lift more than 10 pounds at a time for 6 weeks. Depending on the type of employment, donors may return to work within 2 to 6 weeks.

D.2. Postdonation support

Studies indicate that most donors regard organ donation as a positive experience. That is, they feel good about their decision, experience increased self-esteem, and have a closer relationship with the recipient. But some factors may negatively affect a donor's emotional well-being after donation (e.g., the recipient's outcome, donor complications, degree of donor support available). Although infrequent, some donors have described mild depressive-like symptoms immediately after the surgery. For example, some have reported feeling "forgotten" after the surgery or experiencing a sense of loss (i.e., kidney, short-term bodily functions). Others are not accustomed to feeling pain, feeling ill, or relying on others as they do during their recovery. These feelings usually subside as donor strength and function return.

Donors are aware that they should contact the transplant team and social worker if they experience any emotional distress. However, they may require encouragement from their local physician, if issues are first brought to his or her attention.

E. Donor Financial Issues

Donors do not pay for any of the medical tests or surgery related to kidney donation and, once they are approved, the Transplant Center covers any costs related to potential donor complications. In addition, the Transplant Center's acquisition fee covers the donor's living expenses. Thus, donors should not experience financial hardship as a direct result of donation.

However, some donors do encounter financial problems. If employed, they may be eligible for sick, vacation, or short-term disability benefits (if the donors have coverage and meet employer criteria). Federal employees are eligible for 30 days of paid leave when donating an organ. Some states offer state employees similar benefits of paid leave. In addition, financial grants may be available to help defray donor-related expenses. Donors should discuss these issues with their transplant coordinator or social worker.

Studies indicate that donors do not usually have difficulty obtaining or maintaining health or life insurance following donation. If they do, they are aware to report such problems to the Transplant Center, so measures may be taken to help rectify the situation.

F. Donor Follow-up

As donors are healthy individuals, the required follow-up is usually minimal. The donor should be seen in the Transplant Clinic for an incision check 2 weeks postoperatively and have a creatinine level and urinalysis performed

6 weeks postoperatively. He or she also should receive regular annual medical follow-up appropriate for his or her age.

In addition, donors are advised that they should contact the Transplant Center with any future problems that they think might be related to surgery and/or donation.

CATHERINE GARVEY, RN, BA, CCTC,
AND CHERYL JACOBS, MSW, LICSW

IV. Operative Procedures for Donors and Recipients

A. Laparoscopic Donor Nephrectomy

A.1. History of procedure

Living-donor kidney transplants (LDKT) have been performed successfully since the 1960s via the traditional flank incision. Until the mid-to-late 1990s, open donor nephrectomy, which used the traditional incision, was the primary choice. Consequently, a wealth of accumulated experience helped establish the safety and efficacy of LDKT. In carefully selected individuals, open donor nephrectomy does not adversely affect overall quality of life, long-term kidney function, or longevity. However, such donors do experience significant short-term disability. They undergo a major operation involving a relatively long flank incision, often requiring removal of a portion of the 12th rib. The operation is associated with considerable pain and extensive loss of time from work and other activities. The recovery period usually takes 6 weeks and sometimes longer.

The short-term disability caused by open donor nephrectomy was the impetus to seek an alternative, less invasive method that would result in a smaller incision, less pain, and faster recovery. Laparoscopic donor nephrectomy was first performed in the United States in 1995 and, at the University of Minnesota, in 1997. Currently, more than 90% of our LDKT donors undergo laparoscopic nephrectomy.

A.2. Incision types

Laparoscopic surgery is sometimes referred to as minimally invasive surgery (MIS). It involves the use of small port incisions (usually around 1 cm), which are strategically placed to permit the insertion of surgical instruments. A scope is attached to an external camera to allow the inside of the body to be viewed. The operation is performed from the outside, with the images on the monitor guiding hand movements.

In the case of laparoscopic nephrectomy, the kidney is delivered through an incision just large enough to fit its smallest diameter (usually 2.5 to 3 inches) after it has been methodically freed from its attachments. The incision can be made either vertically in the midline or horizontally below the belt line, at the bikini line (Pfannenstiel incision). The midline incision affords the surgeon an opportunity to insert his or her hand into the abdomen to assist in the operation; it also spares one port incision, thereby resulting in 2 to 3 ports. This approach is called hand-assisted laparoscopic donor nephrectomy. However, with the bikini line incision, the scar is better concealed and the operation may be less painful. The choice of these 2 incisions should be based on the patient's preference, the surgeon's judgment, and other medical factors.

A.3. Early follow-up and outcomes

Most donors who undergo laparoscopic nephrectomy remain in the hospital 2 days after the procedure. The early recovery period (i.e., the first 2 weeks after surgery) involves a gradual return to activities of daily living. At 2 weeks, most donors are able to tolerate mild exercise in addition to regular activities. However, they should wait 4 to 6 weeks before engaging in any strenuous activity, such as heavy (>10 pounds) lifting, pushing, pulling, or climbing.

Studies have shown that laparoscopic donors experience less pain than open nephrectomy donors, as indicated by the decreased use of pain medication (opiates) after the surgery. A shorter hospital stay and faster return to full activity and work also have been documented. Early-to-intermediate follow-up of laparoscopic donors (≤ 5years) has revealed no increase in the risk of complications compared with open donors. However, results from long-term (i.e., 10, 20, and 30 years) follow-up are not available.

A.4. Bowel dysfunction/complications

In contrast to open donor nephrectomy (in which the kidney is approached from behind the abdomen), laparoscopic nephrectomy involves working through the abdominal cavity. Thus, there is a small long-term risk of intestinal obstruction due to scarring within the abdomen. But this risk remains theoretical, and no increased risk of intestinal obstruction has consistently been documented with other types of laparoscopic procedures during the last 20 years. Laparoscopic donors may, however, experience bowel dysfunction (e.g., nausea, bloating, irregular bowel movements) during the first few postoperative days. Such short-term dysfunction usually responds to a combination of bowel rest and laxatives.

A.5. Time until optimal graft functioning

Much has been written about the advantages to the donor of laparoscopy. Yet its effects, if any, on the donated kidney (and recipient) also must be considered. During the early years of laparoscopy (1995-1998), researchers noted that kidneys harvested via laparoscopic nephrectomy took longer before they began to function optimally in the recipient than kidneys harvested via open donor nephrectomy. This delay occurred despite similar graft survival, recipient survival, and rejection rates between procedures.

This delay in the onset of optimal kidney functioning was attributed to several reasons. First, early laparoscopic nephrectomies took considerably longer to perform than open donor nephrectomies. Second, the carbon dioxide insufflation used during laparoscopic nephrectomy increased abdominal pressure. Since the late 1990s, operative times have become shorter, and techniques have been modified to decrease pressure in the abdomen. These and other developments successfully eradicated the delay in the onset of optimal kidney function in the recipient. In fact, results from several studies reported in 2000 and 2001 indicate no difference in this time for kidneys harvested laparoscopically versus by open donor nephrectomy.

A.6. Nephrectomy outcomes at F-UMC

Since December 1997, we have performed about 250 laparoscopic nephrectomies at the University of Minnesota/Fairview-University Medical Center (F-UMC). We analyzed outcomes from our first 150 laparoscopic nephrectomies and compared them to outcomes from 206 open donor nephrectomies performed during the same period. Consistent with other centers, our results indicate that laparoscopic nephrectomy does not adversely affect the time until the onset of optimal function, rejection rates, patient survival, or graft survival (see table below).

NEPHRECTOMY TYPE	OPEN-DONOR	LAPAROSCOPIC	P
Graft survival			
1 year	91%	99%	0.02
2 year	87%	94%	0.02
Patient survival			
1 year	97%	98%	0.3
2 year	95%	98%	0.3

Some centers avoid right-sided laparoscopic nephrectomy due to technical considerations. However, we can remove either the left or the right kidney laparoscopically at the F-UMC. In our analysis, we found no difference in recipient outcomes between those receiving a right or left kidney. We also found that the outcomes of obese and nonobese donors were similar. However, to ensure their own safety, we recommend that overweight donors lose weight and reach a body mass index (BMI) of less than 30 prior to donation. (BMI is calculated from the height and weight of a person. For example, the BMI of a 6-foot, 209-pound person is only 27, compared to 39 for a 5-foot person of the same weight.) Morbidly obese donors (BMI >35) may be ineligible to donate a kidney.

In another study, we assessed the psychological profile and satisfaction of both types of donors. After donation, laparoscopic and open donors had mental health scores higher than those for the average US population. Interestingly, laparoscopic donors were less satisfied with their scars despite having smaller incisions. This may reflect higher expectations from laparoscopic surgery or the use of multiple port incisions. As the small port-site scars fade with time, satisfaction may increase.

In summary, laparoscopic nephrectomy represents a less invasive surgical option than open nephrectomy, offering the kidney donor advantages such as smaller less-visible scars, less postoperative pain, and faster return to normal activities. There are no obvious disadvantages to the recipients. Long-term (10 to 20 years) follow-up data will be available in the next few years and will be vital in determining the future of this procedure. Meanwhile, laparoscopic nephrectomy is gaining in popularity, with more than 90% of kidney donors at F-UMC selecting it.

B. Transplant Operative Procedure

A detailed description of the kidney transplant operative procedure and anesthetic management is beyond the scope of this chapter. However, a basic understanding of the procedure and the intraoperative course is needed to optimize postoperative care and monitor for possible complications.

B.1. Surgical approach

The surgical technique for kidney transplantation has changed very little from the original pelvic operation described in 1951 by Kuss and colleagues. The most common approach used today is the standard pelvic operation, with retroperitoneal placement of the kidney allowing easy access for percutaneous biopsy. Usually, the right iliac fossa is chosen because of the more superficial location of the iliac vein on this side. However, the left iliac fossa should be used when the recipient is a potential candidate for a future pancreas transplant, is receiving a second transplant, or has significant arterial disease on the right side (Fig 1). Another option is to place the kidney in an intraabdominal position through a midline incision. This option is useful when simultaneous pancreatic transplantation is being performed or when a recipient has previously undergone operations on both the left and right iliac veins (Fig 2).

With the standard pelvic operation, the dissection is extraperitoneal. The iliac vessels are identified and assessed for suitability for anastomosis. The internal iliac artery can be used as the inflow vessel, with an end-to-end anastomosis; alternatively, the external iliac artery can be used, with an end-to-side anastomosis. To minimize the risk of lymphocele formation, only a modest length of artery is dissected free, and the lymphatics overlying the artery are ligated. The donor renal vein is anastomosed end-to-side to the external iliac vein.

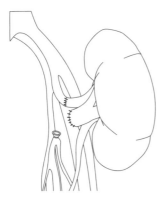

Figure 1: Kidney transplant in the left iliac fossa, with anastomoses to the recipient's internal iliac artery.

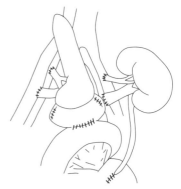

Figure 2: Simultaneous pancreas and kidney transplantation, with the kidney placed in an intraperitoneal position.

After the vascular anastomosis is completed and the kidney perfused, urinary continuity can be restored by a number of different methods. The most common techniques used are a posterior Leadbetter-Politano, an anterior multistitch (Litch), or an anterior single-stitch. Results with the 3 techniques are similar. Regardless of the technique used, the anastomosis must be tension-free and protected by at least a 1-centimeter submucosal tunnel to prevent reflux during voiding.

The transplant operation for larger pediatric recipients (i.e., >20 kg) is similar to that for adults. For smaller recipients, the kidney is usually placed in an intraperitoneal position through a midline abdominal incision; more proximal blood vessels, such as the infrarenal aorta and inferior vena cava, should be used for implantation (Fig 3).

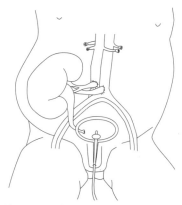

Figure 3: Kidney transplant in an infant recipient. The kidney has been placed in an intraperitoneal position, with anastomoses to the recipient's aorta and inferior vena cava.

B.2. Intraoperative care

Intraoperative care of transplant recipients is not unlike that of other patients undergoing major surgical procedures. To decrease the incidence of acute tubular necrosis (ATN) posttransplant, a liberal hydration policy is employed intraoperatively. Adequate perfusion of the transplanted kidney is important to ensure postoperative diuresis. Central venous pressure (CVP) should be maintained around 10 mm Hg and systolic blood pressure, greater than 120 mm Hg. Maintaining adequate CVP is especially important in smaller pediatric recipients, because reperfusion of the adult-sized kidney graft may divert a significant amount of their blood volume. Administration of mannitol and furosemide just before reperfusion usually helps maximize perfusion of the new kidney.

RAJA KANDASWAMY, MD, AND ABHINAV HUMAR, MD

V. Early Posttransplant Care

A. Immediate Postoperative Care

The immediate postoperative course can range from smooth to extremely complicated. It mainly depends on the recipient's preoperative status as well as the development of any postoperative complications. The care of all transplant recipients involves:

- Stabilization of the major organ systems (e.g., cardiovascular, pulmonary, renal).
- Evaluation of graft function.
- Achievement of adequate immunosuppression.
- Monitoring and treatment of complications directly and indirectly related to transplantation.

The initial postoperative care usually does not need to be performed in an intensive care unit, as most recipients do not require mechanical ventilatory support. The goal is to maintain adequate oxygen saturation, acid-base equilibrium, and stable hemodynamics. This goal can generally be met on a regular surgical ward, with adequately trained nursing personnel.

A.1. Hemodynamic status

Initially, as with all postsurgical patients, hemodynamic stability is assessed via measurement of blood pressure (BP), heart rate, and urine output. Monitoring of the pulmonary wedge pressure is usually not necessary, except perhaps in recipients with underlying myocardial dysfunction. Monitoring of the central venous pressure (CVP) may help guide fluid replacement therapy. Placement of an arterial line is usually unnecessary, but regular, frequent BP monitoring is important. Increased BP may increase the risk of postoperative bleeding and cerebrovascular accidents (stroke), whereas low BP may increase the risk of graft thrombosis or acute tubular necrosis (ATN). Achieving hemodynamic stability is not only important to the recipient's overall status, but also necessary for optimal graft function; hemodynamically unstable recipients will experience poor perfusion of the newly transplanted kidney.

A.2. Fluid and electrolyte management

Careful attention to fluid and electrolyte management is crucial. In general, transplant recipients should be kept euvolemic or slightly hypervolemic. If initial graft function is good, fluid replacement can be regulated by hourly replacement of urine. Half-normal saline is a good solution to use for urine replacement.

Aggressive replacement of electrolytes, including calcium, magnesium, and potassium, may be necessary, especially in recipients undergoing brisk diuresis. Those with acute tubular necrosis (ATN) and fluid overload or hyperkalemia may need fluid restriction and even hemodialysis. Magnesium levels should be maintained above 2 mg/dL to prevent seizures, and phosphate levels should be maintained between 2 and 5 mg/dL for proper support of the respiratory and alimentary tracts. Marked hyperglycemia, which may be secondary to steroids, should be treated with insulin.

Hypotension is unusual early after kidney transplantation. When it does occur, it is usually related to hypovolemia. The appropriate treatment is optimization of the preload and afterload, with use of inotropic agents (e.g., dopamine, dobutamine) only if necessary. Systemic hypertension is more common during the early posttransplant period. If catecholamine-mediated or a side effect of immunosuppressive agents, the hypertension usually responds well to calcium channel blockers. But if it is secondary to fluid overload and accompanied by poor kidney function, dialysis may be necessary.

A.3. Gastrointestinal care

Transplant recipients usually do not require nasogastric suction unless the kidney graft has been placed in an intraperitoneal position. However, some form of prophylaxis for gastrointestinal (GI) bleeding should be maintained, as physiologic stress, coupled with high-dose steroid therapy posttransplant, may lead to gastric erosions and ulcerations. Recipients can usually begin a liquid diet the day after transplantation and then advance to a regular diet as tolerated.

B. Graft Function

A crucial aspect of postoperative care is the repeated evaluation of graft function, which begins intraoperatively, soon after the kidney is reperfused. Signs of good kidney function include appropriate color and texture along with evidence of urine production. Upon the recipient's arrival in the recovery room or transplant ward, clinical signs and laboratory values guide the continuing evaluation of kidney function.

B.1. Indicators and grades of graft function

Urine output is the most readily available and easily measured indicator of graft function. Urine volume may range from none (anuria) to large quantities (polyuria). When using posttransplant urine volume to monitor graft function, the clinician must have at least some knowledge of the recipient's pretransplant urine volume. If an individual was relatively anuric pretransplant but then has normal urine output posttransplant, graft function is evident. Yet if urine volume was significantly high pretransplant, normal urine volume posttransplant does not necessarily mean good graft function. In such situations, the urine output may reflect that of the native rather than the newly transplanted kidney.

Laboratory values commonly used to assess graft function include serum blood urea nitrogen (BUN) and creatinine (Cr) levels. Recipients can be divided into 3 groups based on initial graft function, as indicated by their urine output and serum Cr level:

- *Immediate graft function (IGF):* Recipients with IGF have a brisk diuresis and a rapidly decreasing serum Cr level posttransplant and do not require dialysis. By our center's definition, their serum Cr is less than 3 mg/dL by postoperative day 5. Most living donor kidney recipients and 50% of cadaveric kidney recipients are in this category. Overall, these recipients have better long-term results and a lower risk of rejection than recipients with poor initial graft function.

- *Slow graft function (SGF):* Recipients with SGF have a moderate degree of kidney dysfunction posttransplant, but they are certainly not anuric and do not require dialysis. By our center's definition, their serum Cr is greater than 3 mg/dL by postoperative day 5. About 25% of cadaveric kidney recipients are in this category. Slow graft function is part of the spectrum of types of graft dysfunction encountered posttransplant, representing a milder form of delayed graft function (DGF). The pathophysiology of SGF and DGF is likely similar, and prolonged ischemia plays a significant role. Compared with recipients with IGF, those with SGF are at higher risk for acute rejection. Any episodes of acute rejection have a significant negative impact on long-term graft survival.

- *Delayed graft function (DGF):* Recipients with DGF have posttransplant graft dysfunction that is at the far end of the spectrum. By our center's definition, these recipients have minimal to no urine output posttransplant and require dialysis support. Delayed graft function generally represents an ischemic injury to the kidney, which may have resulted from donor factors (e.g., increased donor age, cardiac arrest), preservation factors (e.g., prolonged cold ischemic time), or recipient factors (e.g., prolonged warm ischemic time, high panel reactive antibody [PRA]). Recipients with DGF generally improve over a matter of days to weeks, as the kidney recovers from the injury. This type of graft dysfunction should be differentiated from other causes of severe kidney dysfunction early posttransplant, such as graft thrombosis, ureteral disruption, or accelerated acute rejection. Like SGF, DGF is associated with an increased risk for acute rejection, which has a significant negative impact on long-term graft survival.

B.2. Assessment and management of low urine output

Decreased or minimal urine output is a frequent posttransplant concern. Assessment of this problem begins by obtaining a brief history of the clinical situation and asking some important questions. For example, was there initially good urine output followed by a sudden decline, or has there been poor urine output since the transplant? The former suggests an acute catastrophic event (e.g., graft thrombosis), whereas the latter suggests delayed graft function (DGF). Another important question relates to the type of transplant. Was this a cadaveric transplant, with associated risk factors for graft dysfunction (e.g., older donor age, prolonged ischemic time), or was this a living donor transplant? Poor or no urine output in the former case would likely be due to DGF, which would be uncommon in the latter situation.

Once a brief history has been obtained, the recipient is examined. Volume status and fluid balance are assessed to try to determine if the recipient is hypervolemic, euvolemic, or hypovolemic. The Foley catheter also is checked to rule out occlusion by clots or debris. The type of intervention depends on the cause of the graft dysfunction. If the Foley catheter is occluded, it should be irrigated. If the recipient is hypovolemic, an intravenous fluid bolus is indicated. If the recipient is euvolemic or hypervolemic, intravenous diuretics should be administered.

If the above interventions are not successful, then further diagnostic studies should be conducted to try to determine the cause of the poor urine output. For example, a Doppler ultrasound study should be performed to determine flow to the graft and rule out thrombosis. A renal scan also will help assess flow to the kidney graft and might rule out urinary leakage or obstruction. Eventually, kidney biopsy may be necessary to evaluate the possibility of an early episode of acute rejection.

C. Immunosuppression

One important aspect of early posttransplant care is immunosuppression, which is typically divided into the following 2 phases:

- *Induction immunosuppression:* Induction therapy refers to the drugs given immediately posttransplant to induce immunosuppression. At our center, most recipients begin a 4-drug protocol consisting of: 1) a calcineurin inhibitor (cyclosporine [CsA] or tacrolimus), 2) a purine synthesis inhibitor (mycophenolate mofetil [MMF] or azathioprine [AZA]), 3) a corticosteroid (prednisone or methylprednisolone), and 4) a polyclonal antilymphocyte agent. Currently, we use a steroid-avoidance regimen for most of our recipients, i.e., they usually receive a corticosteroid for only 4 to 5 days before it is discontinued. In recipients with slow graft function (SGF) or delayed graft function (DGF), the dose of the calcineurin inhibitor (which can be nephrotoxic) should be limited or the drug temporarily withheld until kidney function improves.

- *Maintenance immunosuppression:* Maintenance therapy refers to the drugs given to maintain immunosuppression once recipients have recovered from the operative procedure. At our center, we generally tend to decrease the level of immunosuppression as the time posttransplant lengthens and as the risk for rejection decreases. Most commonly, the dose of the calcineurin inhibitor is reduced and the dose of MMF or AZA slightly decreased at 3 to 6 months posttransplant. As stated above, most of our recipients now receive steroids for only the first 4 to 5 days posttransplant, so steroids are not part of our maintenance protocol. The target levels for the calcineurin inhibitor decrease as the time since transplantation lengthens. Higher levels are targeted during the first 2 to 3 months posttransplant, when risk for acute rejection is highest.

Section VI provides detailed information about immunosuppressive drugs, including their mechanisms of action, pharmacokinetics, side effects, dosing, and blood level monitoring. Section VII describes current immunosuppressive protocols used at our institution, including the recently developed steroid-avoidance protocol.

D. Surgical Complications

Monitoring for potential surgical complications is critical. Early diagnosis and appropriate intervention are important to minimize their detrimental impact on the graft and the recipient. Potential surgical complications include the following:

D.1. Hemorrhage

Bleeding is uncommon after kidney transplantation. When it does occur, it is usually from unligated vessels in the graft hilum or from the recipient's retroperitoneum. A falling hematocrit level, hypotension, and/or tachycardia should alert the clinician to the possibility of bleeding. If a drain is present, it may provide visible evidence of bleeding. Surgical exploration is seldom required, because the bleeding often tamponades. However, ongoing transfusion requirements, hemodynamic instability, and compression of the kidney by a hematoma are all indications for surgical reexploration. Often, no major bleeding vessel is identified at relaparotomy, and evacuation of the hematoma is performed.

D.2. Vascular complications

Vascular complications can involve the donor vessels (e.g., renal artery thrombosis, renal vein thrombosis), the recipient vessels (e.g., iliac artery thrombosis, pseudoaneurysms, deep venous thrombosis), or both. Renal artery thrombosis (RAT) usually occurs early posttransplant; it is an uncommon event, with an incidence of less than 1%. However, it is a devastating complication, usually resulting in graft loss.

Renal artery thrombosis typically is caused by a technical problem, such as intimal dissection or kinking or torsion of the vessels. Risk factors include hypotension, multiple renal arteries, and unidentified intimal flaps. Other causes of RAT include hyperacute rejection, unresponsive acute rejection, and a hypercoagulable state. Patients with RAT typically present with a sudden cessation of urine output. The diagnosis is easily made with color flow Doppler studies. Urgent thrombectomy is indicated, but most grafts cannot be salvaged and require removal.

Patients with stenosis of the renal artery, a late complication, present with hypertension or evidence of graft dysfunction. Doppler studies constitute a good screening examination, with high sensitivity (88%) and specificity (100%) for this condition. First-line treatment for renal artery stenosis involves interventional radiologic techniques; surgery is reserved for stenosis that does not respond to these methods.

Arterial complications that affect recipient vessels are much less common but can be equally devastating. Early events, such as iliac artery thrombosis, can be limb threatening. Late complications, such as formation of a pseudoaneurysm or fistula, can lead to significant hemorrhage. Risk factors include underlying peripheral vascular disease (PVD), deep infections, and type I (insulin-dependent) diabetes. Prompt surgical exploration with balloon thrombectomy is essential to salvage the limb and prevent long-term sequelae from these complications.

Renal vein thrombosis is not as common as its arterial counterpart, but, again, graft loss is the usual end result. Its causes include angulation or kinking of the vein, compression by a hematoma or lymphocele, anastomotic stenosis, and extension of an underlying deep venous thrombosis (DVT). Again, a Doppler study is the best means of diagnosing this complication. Urgent thrombectomy is rarely successful and nephrectomy is usually required.

Venous thromboembolic complications that affect the recipient vessels (DVT and pulmonary embolism [PE]) are not uncommon. The incidence of DVT is close to 5% and that of PE, 1%. Identified risk factors include recipient age older than 40 years, diabetes, and a history of DVT. For recipients with these risk factors, prophylactic treatment with low-dose heparin is recommended.

D.3. Urologic complications

Urinary tract complications, manifesting as leakage or obstruction, occur in about 2% to 10% of kidney transplant recipients. The underlying cause is generally ischemia due to poor blood supply to the transplant ureter, and leakage usually occurs from the anastomotic site. Undue tension, created by a short ureter or direct surgical injury, is another cause of urologic complications.

Patients with urinary leakage usually present early (before the 5th posttransplant week); symptoms include fever, pain, swelling at the graft site, increased creatinine level, decreased urine output, and cutaneous urinary drainage. A hippurate renal scan can confirm the diagnosis. Early surgical exploration with ureteral reimplantation is usually indicated, though small leaks may be managed by percutaneous nephrostomy and stent placement with good results.

Obstruction can occur early or late. Early obstruction may be due to edema, blood clots, hematoma, or kinking. Late obstruction generally reflects scarring and fibrosis due to chronic ischemia. Patients usually present with an increase in their serum creatinine level. Ultrasonography, looking for hydronephrosis, is a good initial diagnostic test. A lasix renogram is useful in less obvious cases, but percutaneous nephrostogram is the most specific diagnostic test. Initial treatment with percutaneous transluminal dilatation (PTD), followed by placement of an internal or external stent, has yielded good results.

Another potential urinary complication is hematuria. Mild hematuria is not infrequent and is usually observed during the first 12 to 24 hours posttransplant. In most patients, it usually resolves spontaneously. More extensive bleeding may result in retained blood clots and urinary tract obstruction, which is the most common cause of sudden cessation of urine output immediately posttransplant. Continuous bladder irrigation will usually restore diuresis; if unsuccessful, cystoscopy may be necessary to evacuate the clot and cauterize the source of the bleeding.

D.4. Lymphoceles

Lymphoceles are collections of lymph in the recipient that generally result from cut lymphatic vessels. Lymphoceles usually do not occur until at least 2 weeks posttransplant, and their incidence ranges from 0.6% to 18%. Symptoms are generally related to the mass effect and compression of nearby structures (e.g., ureter, iliac vein). Although ultrasound can confirm the presence of a collection of fluid, percutaneous aspiration may be necessary to rule out another type of fluid collection (e.g., urinoma, hematoma, abscess).

The standard surgical treatment of a lymphocele involves creation of a peritoneal window; this allows drainage of the lymphatic fluid into the peritoneal cavity, where it can be absorbed. Either a laparoscopic or an open approach may be used. Another therapeutic option is the percutaneous insertion of a drainage catheter, with or without sclerotherapy; however, this option is associated with some risk of recurrence or infection. A combination of the two methods may be used; the lymphocele is initially drained percutaneously via a drainage catheter and then sclerotherapy is attempted. If the lymphocele continues to drain, recurs, or is not amenable to initial percutaneous drainage, a laparoscopic or open peritoneal window is created instead.

D.5. Wound infections

Wound infections are fairly infrequent after kidney transplantation, with an incidence of only 1% to 2%. They may be superficial or deep to the fascia. Deep infections are generally related to complications such as urinary leakage. Superficial infections are more common than deep infections and reflect contamination from skin organisms or from contaminated urine (when the bladder anastomosis was performed).

Deep infections are treated with drainage—intraoperative or percutaneous—and, usually, antibiotics too. Superficial infections are often treated via opening of the surgical wound and allowing it to heal by secondary intention; antibiotic therapy is usually unnecessary unless the recipient has significant cellulitis or systemic symptoms.

E. Medical Complications

Medical problems unique to kidney transplant recipients are usually related to infections or graft dysfunction secondary to rejection or drug toxicity.

E.1. Rejection

The 4 types of clinical rejection are hyperacute rejection, accelerated rejection, acute rejection (AR), and chronic rejection (CR). Only the first 3 types are seen during the early posttransplant period; the last type (CR) remains the most frequent cause of late graft failure. Hyperacute and accelerated rejection occur very early after transplantation and reflect host anti-donor presensitization. With current cross-match techniques, these 2 types of rejection are relatively rare. However, AR is more common, now affecting about 15% of transplant recipients. Most prevalent in the first few months posttransplant, AR is unusual beyond the first year. Late episodes of AR should raise clinical suspicion of noncompliance with medication regimens.

With current immunosuppression protocols, symptoms such as fever, graft tenderness, malaise, and oliguria are unusual with AR. The most common manifestation is an asymptomatic rise in the serum creatinine (Cr) level. The previously discussed surgical complications, as well as medical causes of increased Cr (e.g., dehydration, infection, calcineurin-induced nephrotoxicity), must be ruled out. Physical examination, routine biochemistry tests, cyclosporine or tacrolimus blood level determination, and a Doppler ultrasound study will usually provide a definitive diagnosis. However, the diagnosis of AR is ultimately best established via kidney biopsy. Treatment is based on the severity of the rejection, degree of dysfunction, and previously administered immunosuppressive agents. Therapeutic options include a course of high-dose steroids or antilymphocyte preparations (Thymoglobulin or OKT3).

E.2. Cardiac complications

The incidence of cardiac complications posttransplant depends on the recipient's underlying disease, cardiac history, and the level of graft function. Recipients with diabetes, hypertension, or significant coronary disease are more likely to develop cardiac complications and may require perioperative intensive care unit monitoring. Correction of uremia by immediate functioning of the transplanted kidney improves the cardiac index, stroke volume, and ejection fraction.

Myocardial infarction is uncommon, occurring most frequently in recipients with preexisting risk factors. Pericarditis may occur early posttransplant, but its incidence is only 1% to 3%. Pericarditis usually occurs secondary to uremia, but other causes include infection (e.g., cytomegalovirus) and certain medications. Pericardiocentesis is mandatory if a recipient develops cardiac failure, hypertension, or cardiac tamponade.

E.3. Pulmonary complications

Most kidney recipients do not require postoperative ventilatory support unless complications such as pulmonary edema or pneumonia develop. Pulmonary edema is usually the result of overly aggressive intraoperative fluid replacement. Treatment involves fluid restriction and diuresis with intravenously administered diuretics followed by hemodialysis, if necessary. Another important cause of pulmonary edema in kidney transplant recipients is an adverse reaction to the monoclonal anti-T cell treatment (OKT3) used for induction or anti-rejection therapy.

Pneumonia remains one of the most common posttransplant infections, with an incidence of 10% to 25%. An aggressive approach to diagnosis is required, usually including bronchoscopy to determine the pathogen(s) involved. If respiratory failure ensues, temporary ventilatory support may be necessary. In addition, appropriate antimicrobial or antiviral agents should be administered, and immunosuppression should be reduced or discontinued.

E.4. Metabolic complications

Hyperkalemia is a frequent perioperative problem. It can develop in recipients with acute tubular necrosis (ATN) or in those with poor graft function secondary to acute or chronic rejection. A potassium-binding ion-exchange resin (e.g., Kayexalate) can be administered to recipients who can tolerate slow correction of serum potassium levels; those requiring rapid correction should receive intravenous glucose and insulin. Transplant recipients who develop hyperkalemia due to poor graft function may require dialysis.

High-output diuresis immediately following transplantation may result in hypokalemia and requires appropriate potassium replacement therapy. Other less frequent abnormalities seen with high-output diuresis include hypomagnesemia and hypophosphatemia.

E.5. Infectious complications

Infections are by far the most common posttransplant problem. Associated morbidity and mortality have decreased in recent years due to improved methods of prophylaxis and early detection, the development of new drugs, and more aggressive treatment. Yet infections remain one of the leading causes of death, both early and late posttransplant. The risk of infection is higher in older recipients, diabetic recipients, and in those status-post multiple sequential episodes of anti-rejection therapy.

E.6. Gastrointestinal complications

The incidence of posttransplant gastrointestinal (GI) complications is 5% to 25%. Peptic ulcer disease (PUD) and its associated complications (e.g., bleeding, perforation) are the most commonly encountered problems involving the upper GI tract. However, the routine use of H_2-receptor antagonists, proton pump antagonists, and potent antacids has considerably decreased the frequency of PUD.

The most common lower GI tract complications following kidney transplantation are colon perforation and hemorrhage. Perforation may be due to diverticulitis, ischemic colitis, stercoral ulceration, or fecal impaction; an undetermined form of colitis is a less common cause.

E.7. Neurologic complications

As many as 30% of kidney transplant recipients develop neurologic problems. Causes include pretransplant conditions, the underlying disease, and sequelae of the transplant operation itself. Cerebrovascular events (e.g., infarction, transient ischemic attack [TIA], hemorrhage), albeit rare, are the most frequent complication; their incidence usually peaks during the first few posttransplant months. Seizures are another common central nervous system complication. Infections (e.g., bacterial and fungal meningitis, brain abscess) generally occur beyond the immediate posttransplant period.

ABHINAV HUMAR, MD

VI. Immunosuppression

A. Maintenance Immunosuppression

Table 1 summarizes protocols currently used at the University of Minnesota/Fairview-University Medical Center (F-UMC) for maintenance immunosuppression. Most patients are maintained on a 3-drug regimen, although some patients also receive maintenance corticosteroids (4-drug regimen). The regimens usually include the following:

- A calcineurin inhibitor:
  —Cyclosporine (CsA) microemulsion = Neoral (preferred), Gengraf (preferred generic), or Eon (nonpreferred generic); or
  —Tacrolimus = Prograf
  —Cyclosporine = Sandimmune (transplantations before 1994).

- A purine synthesis inhibitor:
  —Mycophenolate mofetil (MMF) = CellCept (usually) or
  —Azathioprine (AZA) = Imuran (transplantation prior to 1996).

- A corticosteroid:
  —Prednisone (usually) or prednisolone (in pediatric patients).

- An mTOR inhibitor (mammalian target of rapamycin):
  —Sirolimus (rapamycin, Rapamune)

Common immunosuppressive medication side effects and drug interactions are summarized in Table 2. Tables 3 to 7 provide more detailed information regarding drug interactions. Table 8 summarizes information regarding the use of immunosuppressive medications in dialysis patients.

A.1. Use of specific maintenance immunosuppressive medications

A.1.a. Cyclosporine (CsA) (Sandimmune, Neoral, Gengraf, Eon)

A.1.a.(1) Mechanism of action

Cyclosporine binds to an intracellular protein, cyclophilin; the CsA-cyclophilin complex binds to calcineurin, an enzyme vital to the transcription of several T-cell cytokines, including interleukin-2 (IL-2). Inhibition of cytokine transcription results in specific and reversible inhibition of immunocompetent T-cell activation, mainly T-helper (CD4) cells.

In clinical use, CsA inhibits approximately 50% of calcineurin activity. The parent compound is mainly responsible for the drug's immunosuppressive effects; however, certain metabolites also contribute.

A.1.a.(2) Pharmacokinetics

Cyclosporine (CsA) is available as a lipid suspension (Sandimmune) and as a microemulsion (Neoral, Gengraf, Eon). The microemulsion is better absorbed from the gastrointestinal (GI) tract.

Following oral administration of CsA, absorption is variable, incomplete, and dependent on brand formulation (Sandimmune versus Neoral, Gengraf, or Eon), population characteristics, transplant type, time passed since transplant, GI transit time, and coadministered medications (e.g., H_2 blockers). Absorption of Sandimmune is also dependent on bile flow.

Bioavailability of Sandimmune is 30% (range: 2% to 89%) and that of Neoral, Gengraf, and Eon, 43% (range: 30% to 68%).

Cyclosporine is highly bound (90% to 98%) to serum lipoproteins and widely distributed. Elimination is biphasic, with a terminal elimination half-life for CsA of 8.4 to 27 hours.

Cyclosporine undergoes extensive first-pass metabolism in the liver, via the cytochrome P450 3A4 isoenzyme system, and less extensive metabolism in the GI tract and kidneys to yield at least 30 metabolites. These metabolites are mainly excreted in the bile, with only 6% excreted in the urine. (Only about 0.1% of the dose is excreted as unchanged drug in the urine.)

Cyclosporine is not dialyzable. Dosage adjustment is generally unnecessary for patients with renal failure, although dose reduction may reduce nephrotoxicity.

A.1.a.(3) Concentration monitoring

The measured blood concentration of cyclosporine (CsA) depends on the biologic fluid examined (serum versus whole blood) and type of assay (radioimmunoassay [RIA] versus high-performance liquid chromatography [HPLC]).

For the typical patient in our program, the target immediate predose (trough) level during the first 3 months posttransplant is approximately 150 to 200 ng/mL (whole blood, HPLC method). This target level is reduced to >125 ng/mL from 3 to 6 months posttransplant and to >100 ng/mL 6 months after transplantation.

Monitoring of the area under the curve (AUC) of a sample, which may be a better measure of total drug exposure than trough levels, is under investigation.[1]

The use of Gengraf, the first generic alternative to Neoral, is still under investigation. Large studies have shown success in the conversion of stable patients from Neoral to Gengraf. Yet data on the use of Gengraf in new transplant patients are incomplete. Patients with stable kidney function 1 year posttransplant may switch to Gengraf, if desired.

The typical frequency of drug concentration monitoring for CsA is as follows:

- Once on Monday, Wednesday, and Friday during hospitalization or periods of instability.
- Three times a week for the first 4 weeks posttransplant.
- Twice a week for weeks 5 through 12 posttransplant.
- Weekly for 3 to 5 months posttransplant.
- Every other week for months 6 through 8 posttransplant.
- Every third week for months 9 through 12 posttransplant.

After dosage adjustments, we recommend waiting at least 3 to 4 days before rechecking blood levels.

A.1.a.(4) Toxicity

Table 2 summarizes usual side effects of CsA therapy.

Nephrotoxicity occurs in approximately one third of patients taking CsA and may be associated with increased immediate predose (trough) drug levels. It is generally reversible, at least in part, upon dose reduction. The underlying mechanism is renal vasoconstrictive effects of the afferent arterioles. Clinically, nephrotoxicity manifests as fluid retention, dependent edema, hyperkalemia, and hyperchloremia. Chronic use of CsA may result in irreversible renal failure due to glomerular fibrosis. Risk increases with the addition of other nephrotoxic agents.

Hypertension, with at least mild-to-moderate elevations in both systolic and diastolic blood pressures, occurs in 50% of patients. It generally develops within a few weeks to a few months after initiation of CsA therapy.

Neurotoxicity occurs in about 30% of patients but may improve with continued therapy. Signs and symptoms of neurotoxicity include headache, fine hand tremor, numbness, tingling, burning sensations, and increased sensitivity to hot or cold in the extremities. Some patients experience altered perceptions, memory loss, or a "spaced out" feeling. Seizures may develop, particularly in patients receiving high-dose steroid therapy.[2] Severe neurotoxicity, which may be associated with a low serum cholesterol levels, is characterized by white-matter changes visible on cerebral computed tomography (CT) or magnetic resonance imaging (MRI) scans.

Hirsutism occurs in about 30% of patients; it is usually mild and involves the face, arms, eyebrows, and back.

Hyperuricemia may develop in some patients, requiring anti-gout therapy.

Gingival hyperplasia occurs in 10% of patients; it may improve with vigorous oral hygiene to eliminate periodontal infection.

Hepatotoxicity occurs in less than 5% of patients. It is characterized by elevated alanine aminotransferase (ALT)/aspartate aminotransferase (AST), gamma-glutamyltransferase (GGT), and bilirubin (cholestatic jaundice) levels.

A.1.a.(5) Dosage forms

Oral suspension

- Available as 100 mg/mL.
- Available as Sandimmune (olive-oil base) and Neoral (lipid microemulsion).
- The liquid must be accurately measured.
- A glass container should be used to minimize adherence to the container. Styrofoam should not be used.
- To increase palatability, the suspension may be mixed with milk, chocolate milk, or juice (orange) at room temperature.
- It may be taken straight or with a chaser.
- It should not be mixed into baby food or formula.

Capsules

- Available as 25- and 100-mg capsules. (Sandimmune also has 50-mg capsules.)
- Available as Sandimmune (corn-oil base) and as Neoral, Gengraf, or Eon (lipid microemulsion).
- Capsules should remain in the blister pack until ready to use.
- The cost is the same for capsules or liquid.

Intravenous (IV)

- Available as a 50-mg/mL solution.
- Intravenous cyclosporine (CsA) should be administered as a continuous infusion. The IV dose is not equivalent to the oral dose. To calculate the IV dose, divide the total daily oral dose by 3 and then divide by 24 to get the hourly rate.
- Dilute in 5% dextrose (D5W) or normal saline (NS), usually at a 1:1 ratio, but dilute further if necessary.
- A central or peripheral IV site may be used.
- Do NOT draw blood out of the IV port to measure CsA levels if CsA has ever been infused into that line. Cyclosporine may adhere to the tubing and contaminate the specimen. Peripheral venipuncture is preferred.

A.1.a.(6) Drug interactions

See Tables 2, 3, and 6 for drug interactions between cyclosporine (CsA) and other medications.

A.1.a.(7) Clinical pearls

The US Food and Drug Administration (FDA) does not consider Sandimmune to be bioequivalent to Neoral/Gengraf/Eon. Therefore, one should not replace the other.

Erythromycin, azithromycin, clarithromycin, and related medications should be avoided during therapy, as they markedly increase serum cyclosporine (CsA) and tacrolimus levels.

Isoniazid (INH), rifampin, and related drugs markedly decrease CsA and tacrolimus serum levels. If needed, they should be used in conjunction with CsA with close monitoring.

One should avoid withholding doses of CsA or tacrolimus in response to a high serum level, unless the patient is showing clinical signs of severe toxicity.

Serum CsA and tacrolimus levels in hospitalized patients are often out of the desired range for multiple reasons, including decreased dietary calorie and fat intake and variability in the time of blood sampling. Avoid making large dosage adjustments in response to blood levels obtained in hospitalized patients.

Oral Sandimmune should be given with meals. Neoral, Gengraf, or Eon can be administered with or without meals.

Cyclosporine must never be stored in the refrigerator or at a temperature greater than 85°F.

Capsules should remain in the blister pack until they are ready to use. Boxes containing 7 days of pills can be set up with CsA but not for more than 1 week at a time.

Doses should be taken at the same time each day to ensure consistent CsA levels. Missed doses must be made up as soon as possible. If it is close to the time for the next dose, the dose should not be doubled.

Cyclosporine should not be given with tacrolimus; 24 hours should elapse between doses of these agents.

The dose of HMG-CoA reductase inhibitors needs to be reduced in patients receiving CsA, because CsA blocks the metabolism of HMG-CoA.

Meticulous oral care is imperative during CsA therapy to help prevent gingival hyperplasia.

A.1.b. Tacrolimus (FK506, Prograf)

A.1.b.(1) Mechanism of action

Tacrolimus is pharmacologically, but not structurally, related to cyclosporine (CsA). Like CsA, it inhibits the cell-mediated immune response by inhibiting T-cell activation. However, it binds to a different immunophilin than CsA, the FK-binding protein 12 (FKBP12). The tacrolimus-FK-binding protein complex then prevents the elaboration of interleukin-2 (IL-2) and other cytokines.

A.1.b.(2) Pharmacokinetics

Absorption of tacrolimus is variable; the peak plasma concentration is achieved in 1.5 to 3.5 hours. Its bioavailability is 14% to 22%.

Elimination is biphasic, with a terminal elimination half-life of approximately 12 hours. Tacrolimus is extensively metabolized by the cytochrome P450 3A4 isoenzyme system to at least 10 metabolites, including 2 with immunosuppressive effects.

Less than 1% of the dose is excreted unchanged in the urine.

Tacrolimus is highly protein bound (75% to 99%), mainly to albumin, alpha-1 acid glycoprotein, and erythrocytes.

A.1.b.(3) Concentration monitoring

The initial desired whole-blood immediate predose (trough) level of tacrolimus is 8 to 12 ng/mL. After 6 months, the desired target range may be decreased to 5 to 10 ng/mL.

For frequency of drug level monitoring, see section on blood concentration monitoring of cyclosporine [VI.A.1.a.(3)].

A.1.b.(4) Toxicity

Table 2 summarizes usual side effects of tacrolimus therapy.

The adverse reactions of tacrolimus resemble those for cyclosporine (CsA). Treatment with both is associated with a similar incidence of nephrotoxicity. However, tacrolimus is associated with a higher incidence of neurotoxicity and a lower incidence of hypertension.

Although hirsutism and gingival hyperplasia have not been linked to tacrolimus therapy, alopecia has occurred. Tacrolimus also may cause hyperglycemia and diabetes mellitus.

A.1.b.(5) Dosage forms

Capsules

- Available as 0.5-, 1-, and 5-mg capsules.

Compounded suspension

- Available as 1-mg/mL suspension.

Intravenous (IV)

- Available as 5-mg/mL solution; dilute with 5% dextrose (D5W) to a concentration of 5 mg/250 mL.
- Tacrolimus must be given as a continuous infusion.
- Like cyclosporine (CsA), the IV tacrolimus dose is one third of the oral dose. Divide the total daily dose by 3, then by 24 to determine the hourly rate.
- Intravenous tacrolimus is more nephrotoxic than the oral formulation, so use of oral tacrolimus is preferred, whenever possible.

A.1.b.(6) Drug interactions

See Tables 2, 3, and 5 for drug interactions between tacrolimus and other medications.

A.1.b.(7) Clinical pearls

Erythromycin, azithromycin, clarithromycin, and related medications should be avoided in patients receiving tacrolimus, because they markedly increase serum levels of tacrolimus and cyclosporine (CsA).

Isoniazid, rifampin, and related drugs markedly decrease tacrolimus and CsA serum levels. If needed, they should be used with close monitoring.

One should avoid withholding doses of tacrolimus or CsA in response to a high serum level unless the patient shows clinical signs of severe toxicity.

Serum levels of tacrolimus and CsA in hospitalized patients are often out of the desired range for multiple reasons (e.g., decreased dietary calorie and fat intake, variability in the time of blood sampling). Avoid making large dosage adjustments in response to blood levels obtained from hospitalized patients.

Clearance of tacrolimus is via the liver. Therefore, serum tacrolimus levels depend on liver function and may rise rapidly in patients with severe liver dysfunction.

The morning dose should be withheld until blood is drawn to determine the tacrolimus level.

To obtain consistent blood levels, doses of tacrolimus should be administered at the same time each day. Missed doses should be made up as soon as possible. If it is close to the next dosing time, the dose should not be doubled.

Tacrolimus should never be given concomitantly with CsA. Twenty-four hours should elapse between doses of these agents.

A.1.c. Azathioprine (AZA, Imuran)

A.1.c.(1) Mechanism of action

Azathioprine (AZA) inhibits lymphocyte replication and function. It is metabolized in the liver to 6-mercaptopurine, which is converted to the active metabolite, thioinosinic acid. Thioinosinic acid inhibits deoxyribonucleic acid (DNA) synthesis by interfering with synthesis of guanylic

and adenylic acids from inosinic acid, thereby
interfering with cell division of activated lymphocytes.

A.1.c.(2) Clinical pharmacology and monitoring

Although the half-life of azathioprine (AZA) is
approximately 4 hours, the duration of immunosuppression is much longer; therefore, the drug is
administered once daily.

A small amount of AZA is excreted in the urine, and
myelosuppression may increase during renal failure.

The dose of AZA should be adjusted to maintain a white
blood cell count greater than 3000 per mm^3.

Liver function tests should be performed at least yearly.

A.1.c.(3) Toxicity

Table 2 summarizes usual side effects of azathioprine
(AZA) therapy.

Hematotoxicity related to AZA usually manifests as a
dose-dependent leukopenia. However, AZA also can
cause anemia or thrombocytopenia.

Hepatotoxicity occurs in some patients in whom
mycophenolate mofetil (MMF) or cyclophosphamide
may be useful treatment alternatives. Pancreatitis
requires discontinuation of AZA, but it may persist
despite drug discontinuation. Other gastrointestinal side
effects of AZA include nausea and vomiting.

Hair loss, usually temporary, also may occur with AZA
therapy. Rash is usually a sign of an allergic reaction.

A.1.c.(4) Dosage forms

Tablets

- Available as 50-mg scored tablets.

Compounded suspension

- Available as 5-mg/mL suspension.

Intravenous (IV)

- Available in 100-mg vials (diluted to 10 mg/mL).
- The IV dose is half of the oral dose.
- The drug may be further diluted with 5% dextrose (D5W) or normal saline (NS) prior to administration over 30 to 60 minutes.

A.1.c.(5) Drug interactions

See Tables 2 and 4 for drug interactions between azathioprine (AZA) and other medications.

A.1.c.(6) Clinical pearls

Azathioprine (AZA) use has declined since the launch of CellCept in 1995. It is now largely used in some pediatric patients and in adult patients who underwent transplantation prior to 1995. Most adult kidney programs have since switched to mycophenolate mofetil (MMF).

The white blood cell (WBC) count should be closely monitored during AZA therapy. The dose should be withheld if the WBC count is less than 3000 per mm^3.

Allopurinol in combination with AZA can cause severe leukopenia, thrombocytopenia, and anemia. These agents must NOT be given together without close monitoring of the WBC count; in addition, the dose of AZA should be reduced to 25% to 30% of the current dose, and the Transplant Center must be notified.

Intravenous AZA is light sensitive.

Patients must take the entire daily dose of AZA in the evening.

As AZA is dialyzable, the dose should be given after dialysis.

If AZA is not tolerated, MMF may be a suitable substitute.

Missed doses of AZA should be made up as soon as possible. If it is close to the next dosing time, the dose should not be doubled. If more than one dose has been missed, the patient should contact the Transplant Center.

Adverse reactions and side effects may persist after cessation of AZA therapy, especially pancreatitis.

A.1.d. Mycophenolate mofetil (MMF, CellCept)

A.1.d.(1) Mechanism of action

Mycophenolate mofetil (MMF) inhibits late-stage T-cell activation by interfering with purine synthesis. First, the drug is converted to the active metabolite, mycophenolic acid (MPA); this is a reversible, noncompetitive inhibitor of inosine monophosphate dehydrogenase, a key enzyme in the *de novo* purine synthesis pathway. Unlike other cell types, lymphocytes are relatively dependent on the *de novo* pathway for purine synthesis, which accounts for the selective inhibition of lymphocyte proliferation.

Mycophenolate mofetil also inhibits antibody formation and cytotoxic T-cell generation.

A.1.d.(2) Clinical pharmacology and monitoring

Routine serum drug monitoring of mycophenolate mofetil (MMF) is not currently being done. Although some data suggest that pharmacokinetic monitoring of either the trough level or the area under the curve may be beneficial, a commercial assay is not currently available. This circumstance may change in the future when more data are available.[3-5]

A.1.d.(3) Toxicity

Table 2 summarizes usual side effects of mycophenolate mofetil (MMF).

Potential toxicities associated with MMF therapy include hematologic complications (leukopenia, thrombocytopenia), increased risk of infection, and gastrointestinal (GI) side effects. The latter include nausea, vomiting, diarrhea, hemorrhage, and/or ulceration (rarely). In some patients, these side effects can be quite severe.

Birth defects have occurred in animal studies.

A.1.d.(4) Dosage forms

Capsules

- Available as 250-mg capsules.

Tablets

- Available as 500-mg tablets.

Compounded suspension

- Available as a 100-mg/mL suspension.

Intravenous (IV)

- Available as a 25-mg/mL solution.
- The manufacturer recommends administering a dilute solution by slow IV drip over no less than 2 hours.
- The IV dose is equivalent to the oral dose.
- Intravenous administration should be used only when oral or nasogastric administration is not feasible.
- The drug must be diluted in 5% dextrose (D5W), as mycophenolate mofetil (MMF) is not considered to be compatible with other fluids or medications. Other medications should not be administered via the same IV tubing during the infusion of MMF.

A.1.d.(5) Drug interactions

Tables 2 and 5 describe drug interactions between mycophenolate mofetil (MMF) and other medications.

A.1.d.(6) Clinical pearls

The usual dose of mycophenolate mofetil (MMF) is 1 gm per os (PO) twice daily (BID). Studies have shown that African-American transplant recipients require higher doses of immunosuppression. Therefore, the recommended dose of MMF in African-American patients is 1.5 gm PO BID.

Mycophenolate mofetil is considered teratogenic. To limit exposure, the capsules must not be opened, and the tablets must not be crushed. Gloves should be worn while administering the suspension. After administration, the intravenous (IV) tubing and bag containing the MMF must be disposed of according to hospital chemotherapy protocols.

Female patients taking MMF should be counseled regarding birth control. Two forms of contraception are recommended, as well as waiting 3 months after drug discontinuation before attempting conception.

To reduce gastrointestinal (GI) side effects, the total daily dose can be divided into three or four doses. The dose may need to be reduced if GI side effects persist.

Monitor the white blood cell (WBC) count closely, and decrease the dose of MMF if the WBC count is less than 3000 per mm^3.

Severe renal impairment is associated with increased concentrations of the drug's active metabolite, mycophenolic acid (MPA). The dose of MMF should be limited to 1 g twice daily in uremic patients.

Aluminum/magnesium hydroxide-containing antacids and cholestyramine can reduce the bioavailability of MPA.

Mycophenolate mofetil is not removed by dialysis.

Missed doses should be made up as soon as possible. If it is close to the next dosing time, the dose should not be doubled. If more than one dose has been missed, the patient should call the Transplant Center.

A.1.e. Sirolimus (rapamycin, Rapamune)

A.1.e.(1) Mechanism of action

Sirolimus, also known as rapamycin, binds to the FK-binding protein 12 (FKBP12) within target cells. This complex then binds to a regulatory protein mammalian target of rapamycin (mTOR) and inhibits its activation.[6-10] This inhibition of mTOR activation suppresses cytokine-driven T-cell differentiation by inhibiting progression of the cell cycle from G_1 to S.

Whereas sirolimus and tacrolimus share the same binding protein (FKBP12), the two drugs do not compete for binding, and the resulting complexes do not interfere with each other. Therefore, the use of sirolimus and tacrolimus in combination is not antagonistic, as originally proposed.[11]

A.1.e.(2) Pharmacokinetics

Sirolimus is rapidly absorbed from the small intestine. Due to extensive metabolism, sirolimus has a total systemic bioavailability of about 14%.[12]

Sirolimus is metabolized in the gut and liver by the cytochrome P450 3A4 isoenzyme system. The parent drug has more than seven metabolites, which are thought to be inactive; all metabolites are eliminated via the liver.

Sirolimus has a slow elimination rate, with an average half-life of 62 hours. This allows sirolimus to be administered just once daily. It also suggests that loading doses should probably be used to achieve therapeutic concentrations relatively quickly.

A.1.e.(3) Concentration monitoring

Results from several studies indicate that monitoring of the immediate predose (trough) serum concentration of sirolimus is necessary.[13-14] A commercially available assay is under investigation. The laboratory at Fairview-University Medical Center has developed an assay for sirolimus, with lab analysis of sirolimus levels performed on Mondays and Thursdays. Initial experience with sirolimus has demonstrated that serum trough concentrations of 5 to 15 ng/mL are necessary to achieve a therapeutic effect. Signs of toxicity appear to correlate with higher levels.[13] Recommendations regarding monitoring are continuing to evolve as clinical experience accumulates.

A.1.e.(4) Toxicity[15]

Table 2 summarizes usual side effects of sirolimus.

Hypertriglyceridemia and hypercholesterolemia have been reported with sirolimus therapy; their incidence and severity increase with higher doses.

Leukopenia and thrombocytopenia also have been reported; for both, the incidence increases with higher drug doses and severity increases if sirolimus is coadministered with mycophenolate mofetil (MMF). Doses should be adjusted to keep the white blood cell count greater than or equal to 3000 per mm³ and the platelet count greater than or equal to 100 000 per mm³.

Hypokalemia and rash also have been reported with sirolimus therapy.

Sirolimus is not believed to be nephrotoxic. However, use of sirolimus in combination with cyclosporine (CsA) has been linked to increases in serum creatinine. This may be due to increases in serum CsA levels while the patient is taking sirolimus (see Tables 2, 3, and 6).

Nausea and vomiting, although not as severe as with MMF, may occur with sirolimus therapy.

There have been a few case reports of interstitial pneumonitis in renal transplant recipients that may be related to sirolimus therapy.[16] Additional information is needed to fully ascertain the effect of sirolimus on the lungs.

Mouth sores (aphthous ulcers) have been reported with sirolimus therapy; their incidence may be related to dose.

A.1.e.(5) Dosage forms

Tablets

- 1-mg coated tablets; these tablets must not be crushed.

Suspension

- 1 mg/mL, commercially available.
- To administer the suspension, the filled syringe should be emptied into a plastic or glass cup containing 60 mL of water or orange juice; this should be vigorously stirred for 1 minute and then taken immediately. Grapefruit juice, apple juice, or other fluids should not be used. Afterwards, the empty glass should be filled with another 120 mL of water or orange juice; this also should be vigorously stirred and swallowed immediately.

- The suspension may also be taken straight, if desired.

A.1.e.(6) Drug interactions

See Tables 2, 3, and 6 for drug interactions associated with sirolimus.

A.1.e.(7) Clinical pearls[17]

Bottles can be stored for a maximum of 30 days at room temperature; otherwise, they should be kept in the refrigerator at 2° to 8°C (36° to 46°F).

Hyperlipidemia can be substantial with sirolimus therapy, and many patients have required some form of lipid-lowering agent to control serum lipid levels. If HMG-CoA reductase inhibitors or fibrates are needed, patients taking cyclosporine (CsA) and sirolimus together should be closely monitored and instructed to watch for signs and symptoms of rhabdomyolysis (see Tables 3 and 6).

Missed doses should be made up as soon as possible. If it is close to the next dosing time, the dose should not be doubled. If more than one dose has been missed, the patient should contact the Transplant Center.

Sirolimus is not removed by dialysis.

Drugs known to affect CsA or tacrolimus metabolism will probably also affect the metabolism of sirolimus. If medications known to affect CsA or tacrolimus metabolism are administered to a patient receiving sirolimus, dosage adjustment may be necessary.

A.1.f. Corticosteroids (prednisone, prednisolone, methylprednisolone)

A.1.f.(1) Mechanism of action

Corticosteroids have multiple immunosuppressive mechanisms, including alteration of T-cell proliferation, inhibition of cytokine production (including interleukin-2 and interleukin-6), suppression of macrophage function, reduction of adhesion molecule expression, and induction of lymphocyte apoptosis.

The anti-inflammatory activities of these agents include down-regulation of leukotrienes and prostaglandins.

A.1.f.(2) Clinical pharmacology and monitoring

Weight gain occurs in most posttransplant patients.

Blood pressure, electrolytes, and blood glucose levels should be monitored and maintained at the appropriate levels.

A.1.f.(3) Toxicity

Corticosteroid side effects involve many systems such as:

- Endocrine, including Cushing's syndrome, hyperglycemia, steroid-induced diabetes mellitus, and increased appetite.
- Fluid and electrolyte imbalance, including sodium and fluid retention and hypertension.
- Ophthalmologic, including cataracts, exophthalmos, and increased intraocular pressure.
- Psychiatric, including mood alterations and psychosis.
- Gastrointestinal, including ulceration and candidiasis.
- Immunological, including infection, masking of symptoms of infection or other systemic illnesses, and increased white blood cell count.
- Musculoskeletal, including muscle weakness, cramps, aching, and wasting; growth retardation; and osteoporosis with fracture.
- Integumentary, including acne, hair growth, sun sensitivity, delayed wound healing, and diaphoresis.

Table 2 summarizes usual side effects of prednisone.

A.1.f.(4) Dosage forms

Tablets

- Prednisone is available as 1-, 5-, 10-, and 20-mg tablets.

Suspension

- Prednisone is also available as a 1-mg/mL suspension, and prednisolone, as a 3-mg/mL suspension.

Intravenous (IV)

- Methylprednisolone 0.8 mg = prednisone 1 mg.
- Hydrocortisone is used as a stress dose, as needed.

A.1.f.(5) Drug interactions

Tables 2 and 7 summarize drug interactions associated with steroid therapy.

A.1.f.(6) Clinical pearls

Some side effects of corticosteroids are dose related (e.g., psychosis, hyperglycemia, and Cushing's syndrome).

The dosage of steroids will be tapered during the first posttransplant month. Several available protocols are steroid-avoidance or steroid-free protocols. Patients treated according to these protocols may receive only a few days of steroid therapy after transplantation. It is hoped that such steroid-free regimens will reduce or eliminate the above-described litany of side effects. Further research regarding this issue is ongoing.

Antacids can be used if gastritis becomes a problem. The patient should receive ulcer prophylaxis if the daily dose of steroid is equivalent to more than 250 mg of hydrocortisone or more than 40 mg of prednisone.

All patients should be evaluated for prevention of steroid-induced osteoporosis and maintained on calcium (1000 to 1500 mg) plus vitamin D (400 IU). Biphosphonate therapy is often required.

Missed doses should be taken as soon as possible. If it is close to the next dosing time, the dose should not be doubled. If more than one dose is missed, the Transplant Center should be contacted.

All signs and symptoms of infection should be reported immediately.

B. Anti-T cell and T-cell Modulation of Immunosuppression

Anti-T cell and T-cell modulating agents are used in hospital or clinic settings for induction therapy after transplantation or to treat episodes of acute rejection. Anti-T cell compounds work by removing or reducing the number of T cells available to mount a rejection episode. T-cell modulating agents alter the function of the T cell without destroying it.

B.1. Use of specific anti-T cell and T-cell modulating immunosuppressive agents

B.1.a. Anti-thymocyte globulin-rabbit (Thymoglobulin)

B.1.a.(1) Mechanism of action

Thymoglobulin is a purified gamma immune globulin obtained from the immunization of rabbits with human thymocytes. The rabbits produce cytotoxic antibodies directed against antigens expressed on human T lymphocytes. Thymoglobulin is considered a polyclonal antibody, as all the different antibodies produced by the rabbit are combined into one product.

Thymoglobulin's actual mechanism of action is not completely understood; it may involve several mechanisms including: clearance of T cells from the circulation, modulation of T-cell activity, and direct cytotoxic effects on T cells. Depletion of T cells usually occurs within 24 hours of the first dose.[18]

B.1.a.(2) Pharmacokinetics

The initial half-life of Thymoglobulin is around 2 to 3 days. Antigens targeted by Thymoglobulin remain depleted for days after the final dose.

Thymoglobulin clearance decreases with repeated administration. Thymoglobulin serum may be detected in the blood for weeks after the final dose.[19]

Thymoglobulin is not removed by dialysis.

B.1.a.(3) Clinical monitoring

As Thymoglobulin is derived from rabbit serum, patients who receive it will usually develop anti-rabbit antibodies. Studies evaluating the effect of such antibody production have not been completed. Monitoring of lymphocyte counts is recommended during Thymoglobulin therapy to ensure cell depletion.

Our current protocol is to give a full intravenous (IV) dose of 1.25 mg/kg daily when the lymphocyte count is 0.2 per mm^3 or greater. If the lymphocyte count is 0.1 per mm^3, the dose may be cut in half. If the lymphocyte count is 0, the dose may be held. Thymoglobulin is usually not held for longer than 24 hours.

B.1.a.(4) Toxicity

Toxicities related to Thymoglobulin therapy include the following:

- Infusion-related toxicities, including fever, chills, and rigors.
- Respiratory complications, including wheezing, dyspnea, and pulmonary edema (usually during the infusion).
- Hematological toxicities, including leukopenia and thrombocytopenia.
- Infectious complications, including increased risk of cytomegalovirus, bacterial, and fungal infections. Providing additional immunosuppression can lead to the development of posttransplant lympho-proliferative disease (PTLD).
- Phlebitis may occur. Thymoglobulin should be administered via a central line unless the dose has been specifically formulated for administration via a peripheral line.
- Anaphylaxis is rare but can happen, as Thymo-globulin is an animal product. Epinephrine should be administered and supportive measures initiated if anaphylaxis occurs.
- Rash may occur with Thymoglobulin, although this has been rare.

B.1.a.(5) Dosage forms and usual dose

Thymoglobulin is available as a 25-mg dry vial and can be reconstituted with sterile water to a concentration of 5 mg/mL. The dry vials should be stored in the refrigerator; do not freeze. The final solution should have 25 mg of Thymoglobulin per 50 mL of either normal saline or 5% dextrose (D5W).

The usual dose of Thymoglobulin is 1.25-1.5 mg/kg/day. The dose must be filtered with a 0.22-micron filter before administration. The first dose should be infused over a minimum of 6 hours. Subsequent doses can be infused over 4 hours, if tolerated. The dose of Thymoglobulin must be used within 24 hours of being reconstituted.

B.1.a.(6) Drug interactions

Thymoglobulin does not affect metabolism of other medications, nor do other drugs affect its metabolism. However, Thymoglobulin should not be mixed or infused with any other intravenous medications, and the infusion should be via a separate line.

The presence of Thymoglobulin in the circulation may interfere with any rabbit antibody-based immunoassays as well as any cross-match or antibody cytotoxicity assays.[18]

B.1.a.(7) Clinical pearls

Close monitoring during administration of the first dose of Thymoglobulin is vital. The patient's temperature, heart rate, and respiratory rate should be monitored regularly during the infusion.

If a patient starts to develop a reaction to Thymoglobulin, stop or slow the rate of the infusion. If the patient improves, the infusion may be restarted. This usually is only necessary for the first dose.

It is vital that a 0.22-micron filter be used during Thymoglobulin administration, including when the drug is administered during the transplant operation.

It is usually necessary to premedicate patients for Thymoglobulin therapy. We premedicate with 500 mg of intravenous (IV) methylprednisolone before the first dose, along with acetaminophen and diphenhydramine. Doses of acetaminophen and diphenhydramine can be repeated during the middle of the infusion. Subsequent doses of steroids can be timed to premedicate for subsequent doses of Thymoglobulin if necessary.

If rigors are a problem, a small dose of meperidine (25 mg IV) is usually effective.

Do not draw blood for hematologic laboratory tests during infusion of Thymoglobulin, as the white blood cell (WBC) count can significantly decrease during the infusion. The WBC count usually increases soon after the infusion is finished.

Try not to administer blood products at the same time as Thymoglobulin to prevent confusion about the source of a reaction if one occurs.

If necessary, Thymoglobulin can be administered via a peripheral line. In this situation, Thymoglobulin needs to be diluted in 500 mL of normal saline (NS), and hydrocortisone (20 mg IV) and heparin (1000 units) should be added to the bag.

Thymoglobulin use has been associated with an increase in cytomegalovirus (CMV) infections. Therefore, patients receiving Thymoglobulin should also be receiving CMV prophylaxis therapy.

Thymoglobulin is a very expensive medication. Each dose should only be ordered after a daily review of the patient's laboratory values and immunosuppressive protocol.

B.1.b. Muromonab-CD3 (Orthoclone CD-3, OKT3)

B.1.b.(1) Mechanism of action

Muromonab-CD3 (OKT3) is a murine monoclonal antibody directed against the CD3 receptor found on circulating mature lymphocytes. The CD3 antigen on lymphocytes has been shown to initiate intracellular events associated with acute rejection. Once injected, OKT3 either destroys or renders ineffective all of the circulating lymphocytes that express the CD3 receptor. OKT3 can cause T lymphocytes to be removed from the circulation as early as 10 minutes following the injection. It is extremely effective in treating rejection, with 71% of the cases of steroid-resistant rejection among kidney transplant recipients being responsive to OKT3.[20]

B.1.b.(2) Pharmacokinetics

The average half-life of OKT3 is 18 hours; thus, OKT3 is given daily to achieve adequate lymphocyte depletion. As OKT3 is a murine antibody, there is a risk of human anti-mouse antibody (HAMA) formation during or with subsequent OKT3 treatment(s). In such situations, CD3-positive lymphocytes may initially decrease and then slowly increase after a few days, as more OKT3 is rendered ineffective by HAMA.

OKT3 is not removed by dialysis.

B.1.b.(3) Clinical monitoring

Lymphocyte differentials, with measurement of CD3-positive cells, should be monitored closely in patients receiving OKT3. The CD3 counts should drop to less than 10 cells/µl after the first few doses of OKT3. If CD3 counts rise during therapy, human anti-mouse antibody (HAMA) may be present, and the dose should be increased or the drug therapy changed.

Our usual protocol is to check the CD3 level on the third day of therapy and to monitor CD3 counts every other day during the remainder of treatment. If the patient is at high risk for formation of HAMA, CD3 counts should probably be checked daily.

B.1.b.(4) Toxicity

OKT3 therapy is associated with a myriad of toxicities, most related to the destruction or modulation of T lymphocytes. In addition to destroying lymphocytes, OKT3 can augment or induce further cytolytic activity; this leads to the release of multiple endotoxins, including IL-2 and tumor necrosis factor (TNF), in a syndrome described as the cytokine release syndrome.[21]

Symptoms that may be experienced during cytokine release syndrome include:

- Fever (can be high), chills, rigors.
- Nausea, diarrhea, vomiting.
- Chest pain, angina/myocardial infarction, heart failure.

- Hypertension, hypotension (shock), hemodynamic instability.
- Pulmonary edema, dyspnea, wheezing.
- Flu-like symptoms, lack of energy.

Therapy with OKT3 has also been associated with a number of neurologic adverse events including:

- Headache, photophobia.
- Aseptic meningitis (multiple cases).
- Seizures, encephalopathy, coma.
- Blindness, psychosis.

The mechanism underlying these neurologic toxicities is unknown.

Infectious adverse events also may occur with OKT3 therapy including the reactivation of cytomegalovirus (CMV), fungal infections, bacterial infections, and *Pneumocystis carinii* pneumonia (PCP).

Use of OKT3 may increase the risk of posttransplant lymphoproliferative disease (PTLD). This risk may be correlated with the total number of doses received.

Allergic reactions have occurred with OKT3 treatment and may be difficult to differentiate from cytokine release syndrome.

B.1.b.(5) Dosage and dosage forms

A 5-mg dose of OKT3 is usually administered as an intravenous (IV) bolus over 1 to 2 minutes via a peripheral line. There have been several studies documenting the effectiveness of 2.5 mg IV for subsequent doses.[22] Our current policy is to administer additional doses of 2.5 mg IV for a total course of 5-14 doses, depending on the severity of the rejection and the patient response. CD3 counts or OKT3 antibody levels should be monitored if the lower dose is going to be used.

OKT3 is supplied as a 5 mg/5 mL ampule. A half-dose can be split and used for the next day's dose. The drug should be filtered when drawn up into a syringe for injection.

B.1.b.(6) Drug Interactions

There have been no specific drug interactions between OKT3 and other medications reported.

B.1.b.(7) Clinical pearls

OKT3 is a powerful immunosuppressive agent. It should be administered by experienced personnel in a setting in which the patient can be monitored closely.

Premedication is necessary prior to the first dose of OKT3 to help prevent and alleviate symptoms of the cytokine release syndrome. Premedication with a high dose of intravenous (IV) methylprednisolone (8 mg/kg) has been shown to be more effective than use of a lower steroid dose.[23] Our current procedure is to administer 8 mg/kg of IV methylprednisolone (usually 500 mg in an adult) prior to the first dose of OKT3. We also give 650 mg of acetaminophen and 50 mg of IV diphenhydramine (adult doses) 1/2 hour prior to and 2 hours after each administration of OKT3.

To decrease the incidence of pulmonary edema, patients receiving OKT3 should not be more than 3% above their usual weight. If their weight is elevated, diuretic or other fluid-removing therapies should be instituted prior to OKT3 administration. A chest radiograph should be obtained prior to the first dose to rule out preexisting pulmonary edema.

If the patient experiences dyspnea or respiratory distress, supportive care, including nebulizer treatments and oxygen, may be beneficial.

Clinical monitoring during OKT3 therapy is vital to screen for and provide support for the patient if he or she experiences symptoms or signs of cytokine release syndrome. Our current policy is to monitor temperature, blood pressure, heart rate, and respiratory rate every 15 minutes for the first hour, every 30 minutes for the second hour, every hour for the next 4 hours, and every 4 hours afterwards.

The first two doses must be given in the hospital, as some patients may not react to OKT3 until their second dose. Reactions are unusual after the third dose. If the patient is doing well and feeling okay, he or she may be discharged from the hospital and finish the course of OKT3 therapy at the clinic.

B.1.c. Daclizumab (Zenapax)

B.1.c.(1) Mechanism of action

Daclizumab was first in the class of interleukin-2 (IL-2) receptor antagonists. It is a genetically engineered, humanized monoclonal antibody with activity against the CD25 subunit of the activated IL-2 receptor on lymphocytes. The final antibody is comprised of 90% human and 10% murine antibody sequences.

Daclizumab binds with high affinity to the IL-2 receptor, preventing IL-2-mediated activation of lymphocytes.[24] Unlike Thymoglobulin or OKT3, daclizumab does not cause the destruction or removal of circulating lymphocytes.

B.1.c.(2) Pharmacokinetics

Because daclizumab is a humanized antibody, it has extended activity against the interleukin-2 (IL-2) receptor. The average terminal half-life of daclizumab is 20 days, which is similar to that of human IgG. After a routine course of treatment, IL-2 receptor blockade lasted an average of 120 days.[24,25]

Daclizumab is not removed by dialysis.

B.1.c.(3) Toxicity

The main double-blind study that compared daclizumab with placebo revealed that adverse events did not significantly differ between the two groups.[25] To date, cytokine release syndrome has not been associated with daclizumab therapy, nor have long-term toxicities, including posttransplant lymphoproliferative disease (PTLD).

While not yet reported, anaphylaxis is possible with daclizumab administration. If symptoms or signs of anaphylaxis are observed, the infusion should be stopped and supportive measures initiated.

B.1.c.(4) Dosage forms and usual dose

Daclizumab is supplied in glass vials containing 25 mg of drug in 5 mL of solution. The first dose of daclizumab should be administered no earlier than 24 hours prior to the transplant operation. No premedication is required. The recommended dosing schedule is 1 mg/kg IV every 14 days, for a total of 5 doses. The calculated dose is diluted with 50 mL of normal saline and infused over a 15-minute period. The drug for the final infusion must be refrigerated and used within 24 hours of dilution.

B.1.c.(5) Drug interactions

There are no known reports of drug interactions with daclizumab. It has been studied in combination with all of the immunosuppressive and other medications usually used in transplant patients. However, other medications should not be infused in the same line as daclizumab, nor should any other medication be added to the infusion bag.

B.1.c.(6) Clinical pearls

Daclizumab therapy does not require any additional monitoring or premedication.

Due to specific circumstance, some patients may not receive the full 5 doses. Physicians should check with the Transplant Center if they have any questions related to the duration of therapy.

If necessary, subsequent doses of a q-14 day regimen can vary by a day or two to accommodate clinic or patient availability.

Daclizumab is very expensive; the dose and dosing schedule should be verified before the drug is mixed by the pharmacy.

B.1.d Basiliximab (Simulect)

B.1.d.(1) Mechanism of action

Like daclizumab, basiliximab is an interleukin-2 (IL-2) receptor antagonist. It is a genetically engineered, chimeric monoclonal antibody with activity against the CD25 subunit of the activated IL-2 receptor on lymphocytes. The chimeric antibody consists of the entire variable region of the murine monoclonal antibody fused to the constant regions of human IgG.

Basiliximab binds with high affinity to the IL-2 receptor and prevents IL-2 mediated activation of lymphocytes.[26] As with daclizumab, it does not cause the destruction or removal of circulating lymphocytes.

B.1.d.(2) Pharmacokinetics

The average half-life for basiliximab is approximately 7.2 ± 3.2 days. The manufacturer selected a 2-dose regimen, which has been shown to saturate interleukin-2 (IL-2) receptors for about 36 days. A randomized trial that evaluated the 2-dose regimen confirmed that IL-2 receptor saturation lasted for 4 to 6 weeks after administration.[27]

Basiliximab is not removed by dialysis.

B.1.d.(3) Toxicity

In a major comparative trial, cytokine release syndrome was not observed and the reported rate of adverse reactions or malignancies did not differ between patients receiving basiliximab versus placebo.[27]

However, post-marketing reports of cytokine release syndrome have since emerged. In addition, post-marketing reports have described 17 cases of severe acute hypersensitivity reactions, including anaphylaxis. The onset of these reactions was within 24 hours of initial drug exposure.

The manufacturer recommends that the basiliximab infusion be stopped immediately if any severe hypersensitivity reaction occurs. If it occurs with administration of the first dose, the second dose should not be given.

Reported adverse reactions to basiliximab include hypotension, tachycardia, cardiac failure, dyspnea, wheezing, bronchospasm, pulmonary edema, respiratory failure, urticaria, rash, pruritus, and sneezing.[28]

B.1.d.(4) Usual dose and dosage forms

The usual adult regimen for basiliximab therapy is 20 mg IV administered on postoperative days 0 and 4. The first dose should be given within 2 hours of the transplant surgery.

The recommended pediatric regimen for basiliximab therapy (for children and adolescents aged 2 to 15 years) is 2 doses of 12 mg/m^2 each, up to a maximum of 20 mg/dose. The same administration schedule applies.

This product is supplied as a glass vial containing 20 mg of basiliximab; prior to use, the drug is reconstituted with 5 mL of sterile water to a concentration of 4 mg/mL. This reconstituted solution is then further diluted with 50 mL of normal saline (NS) or 5% dextrose (D5W), and the final solution is administered over a 20- to 30-minute interval via a peripheral or central line.

B.1.d.(5) Drug interactions

Basiliximab has been studied in combination with all immunosuppressive and other medications usually used in transplant patients. There are no known drug interactions with basiliximab. However, other drugs should not be added to the infusion bag, nor other intravenous medications administered via the same line, during infusion of basiliximab.

B.1.d.(6) Clinical pearls

Despite the reports of anaphylaxis, no premedication is necessary prior to basiliximab administration.

Basiliximab is very expensive. Ensure that the dose is needed prior to ordering it from pharmacy.

MELISSA KENNEDY, PHARMD, BCPS

References

1. Keown P, Kahan BD, et al. Optimization of cyclosporine therapy with new therapeutic drug monitoring strategies: report from the international Neoral TDM advisory consensus meeting. *Transplant Proc.* 1998;30:1645-1649.

2. Nussbaum ES, Maxwell RE, et al. Cyclosporin A toxicity presenting with acute cerebellar edema and brainstem compression. *J Neurosurg.* 1995;82:1068-1070.

3. Langman LJ, LeGatt DF, et al. Pharmacodynamic assessment of mycophenolic acid-induced immunosuppression in renal transplant recipients. *Transplantation.* 1996;62(5):666-672.

4. Shaw LM, Nicholls A, et al. Therapeutic monitoring of mycophenolic acid: a consensus panel report. *Clin Biochem.* 1998;31(5):317-322.

5. Yamani MH, Starling RC, et al. The impact of routine mycophenolate mofetil drug monitoring on the treatment of cardiac allograft rejection. *Transplantation.* 2000;69(11):2326-2330.

6. Abraham, RT. Mammalian target of rapamycin: immunosuppressive drugs uncover a novel pathway of cytokine receptor signaling. *Curr Opin Immunol.* 1998;10:330-336.

7. Kelly PA, Gruber SA, et al. Sirolimus, a new, potent immunosuppressive agent. *Pharmacotherapy.* 1997;17(6):1148-1156.

8. Morris RE. Rapamycins: antifungal, antitumor, antiproliferative, and immunosuppressive macrolides. *Transplant Rev.* 1992;6:39-87.

9. Sehgal SN. Rapamune (RAPA, rapamycin, sirolimus): mechanism of action immunosuppressive effect results from blockade of signal transduction and inhibition of cell cycle progression. *Clin Biochem.* 1998;31(5):335-340.

10. Dennis PB, Fumagalli S, et al. Target of rapamycin (TOR): balancing the opposing forces of protein synthesis and degradation. *Curr Opin Genet Dev.* 1999;9(1):49-54.

11. McAlister VC, Gao Z, et al. Sirolimus-tacrolimus combination immunosuppression [letter]. *Lancet.* 2000;355(9201):376-377.

12. Zimmerman JJ, Kahan BD. Pharmacokinetics of sirolimus in stable renal transplant patients after multiple oral dose administration. *J Clin Pharmacol.* 1997;37(5):405-415.

13. Kahan BD, Napoli KL, et al. Therapeutic drug monitoring of sirolimus: correlations with efficacy and toxicity. *Clin Transplant.* 2000;14(2):97-109.

14. Kahan BD, Napoli KL. Role of therapeutic drug monitoring of rapamycin. *Transplant Proc.* 1998;30:2189-2191.

15. Groth CG, Backman L, et al. Sirolimus (rapamycin)-based therapy in human renal transplantation: similar efficacy and different toxicity compared with cyclosporine. Sirolimus European Renal Transplant Study Group. *Transplantation.* 1999 Apr 15;67(7):1036-1042.

16. Morelon E, Stern M, et al. Interstitial pneumonitis associated with sirolimus therapy in renal transplant recipients [letter]. *N Engl J Med.* 2000;343(3):225-226.

17. Kahan BD. Efficacy of sirolimus compared with azathioprine for reduction of acute renal allograft rejection: a randomised multicentre study: The Rapamune U.S. Study Group. *Lancet.* 2000 July 15;356(9225):194-202.

18. Thymoglobulin [package insert]. Menlo Park, CA: Sangstat Medical Corporation, 1998.

19. Suthanthiran Gaber AO, First MR, Tesi RJ, et al. Results of the double-blind, randomized, multicenter, phase III clinical trial of Thymoglobulin versus ATGAM in the treatment of acute graft rejection episodes after renal transplantation. *Transplantation.* 1998;66(1):29-37.

20. Hooks, MA, Wade CS, Millikan WJ. Muromonab CD-3: A review of its pharmacology, pharmacokinetics, and clinical use in transplantation. *Pharmacotherapy.* 1991;11(1):26-37.

21. M, Fotino M, Riggio RR, et al. OKT3-associated adverse reactions: mechanistic basis and therapeutic options. *Am J Kid Disease.* 1989;16(5 suppl 2):39-44.

22. Midtvedt K, Tafjord AB, Hartmann A, et al. Half dose of OKT3 is efficient in treatment of steroid-resistant renal allograft rejection. *Transplantation.* 1996;62(1):38-42.

23. Peces R, Urra JM, Escalada P. High-dose methylprednisolone inhibits the OKT3-induced cytokine-related syndrome. *Nephron.* 1993;63:118.

24. Zenapax [package insert]. Nutley, NJ: Hoffmann-la Roche, Inc., 1997.

25. Vincenti F, Kirkman R, Light S, et al. Interleukin-2 receptor blockade with daclizumab to prevent acute rejection in renal transplantation. *New Engl J Med.* 1998;338(3):161-5.

26. Novartis Pharmaceuticals. Basiliximab (Simulect) product monograph. East Hanover, New Jersey, May 1998.

27. Nashan, B, Moore R, Amlot P, et al. Randomised trial of basiliximab versus placebo for control of acute cellular rejection in renal allograft recipients. *Lancet.* 1997;350:1193-1198.

28. Bess AL, Cunningham SR. Novartis personal communication. October 6, 2000.

VII. Current Immunosuppressive Protocols Used at F-UMC

A. Evolution of Protocols

Our immunosuppressive protocols have evolved as new immunosuppressive drugs have been introduced and new studies of efficacy have been conducted. In the 1970s, all transplant recipients were treated with a polyclonal antibody, prednisone, and azathioprine. When cyclosporine was introduced in the 1980s, we began using triple therapy (cyclosporine, prednisone, and azathioprine) for living-donor transplant recipients and sequential therapy (polyclonal antibody, prednisone, and azathioprine at transplant with delayed introduction of cyclosporine) for cadaveric transplants. Analysis of our data revealed that living-donor transplant recipients had more rejection episodes than cadaveric transplant recipients. Therefore, we returned to the continued use of polyclonal antibody for all transplant recipients.

During the 1990s, the Food and Drug Administration (FDA) approved a number of new immunosuppressive drugs. We have added these to our immunosuppressive armamentarium. Having multiple choices of immunosuppressive agents available offers several advantages. For example, if a recipient develops a drug-specific complication, that drug can be stopped and a new drug with similar efficacy but a different side effect profile can be substituted.

B. Development of Steroid-free Immunosuppression

One recent major change in our immunosuppressive protocols is the development of a rapid steroid taper after transplantation. As steroids have numerous significant side effects, a number of studies have evaluated late posttransplant steroid withdrawal. For some recipients, steroid withdrawal was successful, but for others, withdrawal resulted in an episode of acute rejection and loss of graft function.

B.1. Steroid-avoidance protocol at F-UMC

It now appears that steroid avoidance (or a very rapid steroid taper) can be done without increasing the risk of acute rejection. In 1999, we initiated our own steroid-avoidance protocol in low-risk patients—first living-donor transplants with immediate graft function. The following table summarizes the drugs and dosage regimens included in this protocol:

Drug	Dosage regimen
Anti-thymocyte globulin	5 doses, with the first dose given intraoperatively
Solu-Medrol	500 mg, intraoperatively
Prednisone	1 mg/kg on POD #1 0.5 mg/kg on POD #2 and 3 0.25 mg/kg on POD #4 and 5 0 thereafter
Cyclosporine (Neoral)	4 mg/kg BID to achieve blood levels (by HPLC) of 150-200 ng/mL for the first 3 months
Mycophenolate mofetil (CellCept)	1 gm BID

BID: twice daily; HPLC: high-performance liquid chromatography; POD: postoperative day

In terms of outcomes, patient survival and graft survival at 1 year were both 98% in this group of patients. Furthermore, only 13% of the patients experienced acute rejection.

Because of the success of this study, we currently use the steroid-avoidance protocol *for all first and second transplant recipients.* The only exceptions are recipients who are already receiving prednisone at the time of transplantation or those who require prednisone for management of their primary disease. These patients undergo the same steroid taper but are started on 5 mg of prednisone per day on postoperative day 6.

To date, we have had more than 250 recipients take part in our steroid-avoidance protocol and the early data are exciting. We have not seen an increase in rejection compared to when we routinely used steroids. And the recipients are spared steroid-related side effects.

B.2. Continuing research of steroid-avoidance protocols

As described above, a rapid steroid taper has become a routine procedure for all first and second transplant recipients. We are currently investigating whether there is a specific combination of immuno-suppressive agents that offers better short- and/or long-term outcomes when steroids are avoided.

Our institutional review board (IRB) has approved our research protocol. All first and second transplant recipients who provide informed consent to participate in the study receive an identical combination of polyclonal antibody and steroids (as described above). Either cyclosporine and mycophenolate mofetil (CellCept) or tacrolimus (Prograf) and sirolimus (rapamycin) are used for maintenance immunosuppression in these patients.

ARTHUR MATAS, MD

VIII. Posttransplant Follow-up and Care

With the use of new, effective immunosuppressive medications, the rates of acute rejection and early graft failure have declined dramatically in the last 10 to 15 years. Unfortunately, the rate of late graft failure has not declined as rapidly as that of early graft failure. Leading causes of late allograft failure include death with a functioning allograft, chronic allograft nephropathy, acute rejection (often from noncompliance with treatment), and recurrence of the underlying kidney disease. Major causes of death include cardiovascular disease (CVD), cancer, and infection. Many posttransplant complications can be prevented through careful monitoring and prophylaxis.

A. General Approach to Posttransplant Patient Care

There is at least indirect evidence that close, long-term monitoring of patients after kidney transplantation improves outcomes. The best system for posttransplant patient monitoring is one that optimally coordinates care between the referring nephrologist and the Transplant Center. The referring nephrologist provides first-line care, including preventive care. The Transplant Center provides back-up care as well as monitoring of allograft function, immunosuppression, and related complications.

Optimal care requires close communication between the patient, the referring nephrologist, and the Transplant Center. Each patient at the Transplant Center is assigned to and followed-up by a transplant nephrologist, a surgeon, and a nurse coordinator. In addition, a transplant PharmD assists in the monitoring of immunosuppression and possible drug interactions. A social worker and financial counselor, who specialize in the needs of transplant recipients, are also available when needed.

B. Frequency and Timing of Routine Physician Follow-up Visits

The referring nephrologist represents a "first line of defense" against problems and complications. The Transplant Center provides back-up care and expertise on immunosuppression and complications that may affect graft function. Therefore, routine follow-up visits with physicians alternate between the referring nephrologist's office and the Transplant Center, as follows:

ROUTINE POSTTRANSPLANT FOLLOW-UP VISITS	
Time Posttransplant	**Site**
Postdischarge	Transplant Center
2 Weeks	Primary Physician
2 Months	Primary Physician
3 Months	Transplant Center
6 Months	Primary Physician
12 Months	Transplant Center
Annual Visits	Alternates between Transplant Center and Primary Physician

At the time of hospital discharge, the Transplant Center team (surgeon, nephrologist, and coordinator) schedules at least one follow-up visit to the Transplant Center during the first week after discharge. This immediate postdischarge visit is needed to ensure optimal patient education and adherence to immunosuppressive medication regimens as well as to obtain baseline outpatient measurements. These measurements include the glomerular filtration rate (GFR), determined via an iohexol plasma clearance technique, and absorption profiling of the major immunosuppressive medications (see later in section). This visit is also designed to ensure that the referring nephrologist receives the necessary information for the patient's first posttransplant visit with the referring nephrologist, which is usually scheduled for about 2 weeks postdischarge. Occasionally, if there are surgical or medical complications, the patient will return to the Transplant Center for additional follow-up visits before returning home.

The frequency of early posttransplant visits depends on whether there are any complications. Generally, patients are seen frequently during the first few months, when the incidence of complications is high. However, maintaining contact with the Transplant Center, even during the very late posttransplant period, is necessary to prevent complications and encourage long-term compliance with immunosuppressive medication regimens. Data related to other fields of medicine suggest that frequent encounters between the patient and provider facilitate adherence to therapies. Results from some studies even suggest that patients dislike long intervals between visits and that such gaps foster uncertainty about the status of the allograft.

C. Frequency and Timing of Nonphysician Visits and Laboratory Checks

In addition to routine surveillance via scheduled physician visits, patients undergo frequent assessment of vital signs, body weight, and laboratory values to monitor for acute changes in graft function and other complications. In general, these visits are frequent during the first 6 posttransplant months, when the incidences of allograft dysfunction and other complications are high. The frequency of these assessments diminishes as the time since transplantation increases. The following table summarizes the frequency of these visits and parameters assessed:

ROUTINE POSTTRANSPLANT FOLLOW-UP VISITS

Parameter	Day 7[a]	Wks 1-4	Mo 2	Mo 2-3	Mo 3[a]	Mo 3-6	Mo 6	Mo 6-12	Mo 12[a]	Mo >12	Each Year[b]
BP-Weight	√	3/wk	√	2/wk	√	1/wk	√	1/mo	√	1/mo	√
Creatinine	√	3/wk	√	2/wk	√	1/wk	√	1/mo	√	1/mo	√
Hemogram	√	3/wk	√	2/wk	√	1/wk	√	1/mo	√	2/yr	√
Platelets	√	3/wk	√	2/wk	√	1/wk	√	1/mo	√	2/yr	√
Na, K, Cl, CO_2	√	3/wk	√	2/wk	√	1/wk	√	1/mo	√	2/yr	√
Glucose	√	3/wk	√	2/wk	√	1/wk	√	1/mo	√	2/yr	√
Trough levels[c]	√	3/wk	√	2/wk	√	1/wk	√	1/mo	√	2/yr	√
Ca, Phos, Mg	√	1/wk	√		√		√		√		√
BUN	√		√		√		√		√		√
Albumin	√		√		√		√		√		√
Hgb$_{A1C}$	√		√		√		√		√		√
Liver panel[d]	√		√		√		√		√		√
Lipid profile[e]	√		√		√		√		√		√
Spot urine ACR	√				√				√		√
AUC	√				√				√		√[f]
GFR					√				√		√[f]

Checkmarks indicate items obtained at that time, and numbers indicate interval frequencies at which items are obtained.

[a]Visits at the Transplant Center.

[b]Alternate annual visits between the Transplant Center and the referring nephrologist.

[c]Level of cyclosporine or tacrolimus drawn 12 hours after the last dose.

[d]Aspartate and alanine aminotransferases, alkaline phosphatase, direct and total bilirubin.

[e]Fasting total cholesterol, high-density lipoprotein cholesterol, low-density lipoprotein cholesterol, and triglycerides.

[f]Obtained every other year at the Transplant Center.

Abbreviations: Mo, month; wk, week; BP, blood pressure; BUN, blood urea nitrogen; Na, sodium; K, potassium; Cl, chloride; CO_2, total carbon dioxide; yr, year; Ca, calcium; Phos, phosphorus; Mg, magnesium; ACR, albumin-to-creatinine ratio; AUC, area under the concentration-time curve for cyclosporine, tacrolimus, and mycophenolic acid; GFR, glomerular filtration rate

After 6 months, the serum creatinine level is measured monthly for the duration of follow-up, so any episodes of acute rejection can be detected and treated. These frequent creatinine checks, even late after transplantation, serve as a constant reminder to the patient that the allograft will be rejected without appropriate care. That is, these measurements enhance compliance with immunosuppressive medication regimens. Laboratories are asked to send results to both the referring nephrologist and the Transplant Center (usually via telefax) on the same day that the blood is drawn. However, we also ask patients to obtain these results and to "know your creatinine." Patient participation in the monitoring of serum creatinine is an additional fail-safe mechanism to ensure that changes are detected quickly, and it also encourages compliance with medications.

D. Measuring the Glomerular Filtration Rate

Two of the most important components of long-term care for kidney transplant recipients are the measurement of graft function and the monitoring of immunosuppressive drug therapy.[1] Measuring the glomerular filtration rate (GFR) is the only proven, clinically effective method for monitoring chronic changes in kidney allograft function. Although monitoring acute changes in serum creatinine levels is useful for detecting acute rejection, serum creatinine is an unreliable marker of chronic changes in the GFR.[2-4] Assessing the GFR via a more accurate method provides valuable information about the true level of glomerular filtration in an individual patient.

Knowing the true GFR in transplant recipients offers a number of advantages. For one, it helps in dosing of medications that are excreted by the kidney. Monitoring changes in the GFR also helps guide decisions regarding immunosuppressive therapy. Finally, as the GFR is an important prognostic indicator, knowing the true GFR in a patient with poor graft function assists planning for a return to dialysis or retransplantation.

A number of studies have shown that measuring the decline in blood levels after the intravenous injection of an inert marker (e.g., iohexol or iothalamate) is a simple and reliable way of estimating the GFR.[5,6] Most studies suggest that a limited sampling strategy—in fact, a single blood sample—can be used to reliably estimate the GFR.[7-10] However, some investigators have reported that the single-sample method is less accurate than multiple-sample techniques.[11] A reasonable compromise between precision and clinical utility is to obtain two plasma samples after injection of iohexol. The timing of these samples may depend on the estimated GFR, so patients with a higher or lower estimated GFR (based on the Cockcroft-Gault formula) need earlier or later sampling times, respectively. However, a reasonably accurate GFR measurement can be obtained within 6 hours (i.e., during a same-day clinic visit) in patients with an estimated GFR greater than or equal to 20 mL/min.

E. Screening for Proteinuria

Periodic screening for proteinuria is another important facet of monitoring allograft function. The incidence of persistent proteinuria posttransplant is 10% to 25%.[1] The most common causes of proteinuria are chronic allograft nephropathy and recurrent or *de novo* glomerulonephritis.[1] Proteinuria itself may cause renal injury. Thus, it is possible that the often-reported clinical association between proteinuria and poor outcomes could be due to the injurious effects of proteinuria per se. Results from a number of studies in the general population suggest that proteinuria is an important risk factor for cardiovascular disease.[12-14] An albumin-to-creatinine ratio (ACR) provides a reasonably accurate assessment of albumin excretion. A ratio of 30 to 300 mg/g indicates microalbuminuria, whereas higher levels are indicative of more severe glomerular damage.[15]

F. Monitoring Blood Levels of Immunosuppressive Agents

F.1. Cyclosporine levels

A growing body of evidence suggests that monitoring the cyclosporine (CsA) area under the concentration-time curve over 12 hours (AUC_{12}), or "absorption profiling," more reliably predicts acute rejection and CsA toxicity than monitoring 12-hour trough levels. A number of studies have also shown that with a microemulsion preparation of CsA, the AUC_{12} can be estimated using a limited-sampling strategy.[16-20] The International Federation of Clinical Chemistry/International Association of Therapeutic Drug Monitoring and Clinical Toxicology has recently acknowledged the utility of 2-hour post-dose (C2) and other limited-sampling strategies for estimating AUC_{12}.[21] Exactly when to obtain the first AUC_{12} estimate is unclear, although results from a recent multicenter study suggest that AUC_{12} estimates obtained during the first 14 days posttransplant already correlate with early acute rejection episodes.

F.2. Tacrolimus levels

Traditionally, 12-hour drug trough levels have been used to adjust the dose of tacrolimus. At least one retrospective study correlated 12-hour trough levels measured during the first posttransplant month with the subsequent occurrence of acute rejection.[22] However, recent data from liver transplant recipients suggest that obtaining additional drug levels, to better assess tacrolimus absorption, may reduce intrapatient variability and thereby improve monitoring.[23] Unfortunately, there exist few studies to define the best approach for measuring tacrolimus absorption to maximize its efficacy and minimize its toxicity.[21]

F.3. Mycophenolate mofetil levels

Mycophenolate mofetil (MMF) is rapidly metabolized to mycophenolic acid (MPA). Recent studies have suggested that the MPA area under the concentration-time curve over 12 hours (AUC_{12}) is more closely associated with clinical efficacy than 12-hour trough levels.[21,24,25] In addition, preliminary data suggest that limited-sampling strategies may be effective in estimating the AUC_{12} of MPA.[25,26] In particular, one study demonstrated the feasibility of obtaining simultaneous cyclosporine (CsA) and MPA AUC_{12} estimates.[25]

F.4. Sirolimus levels

There is a clear relationship between both the efficacy and toxicity of sirolimus and 12-hour trough drug concentrations.[21] The half-life of sirolimus is approximately 60 hours, and unlike the other immunosuppressive agents, there appears to be a good correlation between 24-hour trough levels and the sirolimus area under the concentration-time curve over 24 hours.[27,28] Therefore, 24-hour trough levels are probably adequate for monitoring sirolimus therapy.

G. Monitoring for Posttransplant Complications

G.1. Hematological complications

Hemoglobin levels, hematocrits, and white blood cell counts should be measured frequently posttransplant (see table in VIII.C.). Anemia and leukopenia are common, especially early after transplantation, and often result from treatment with immunosuppressive agents (e.g. mycophenolate mofetil, sirolimus). Leukopenia is more common in patients from whom corticosteroids have been withdrawn. Erythrocytosis may be seen in as many as 10% of transplant recipients, and it often responds to treatment with angiotensin-converting enzyme inhibitors. Thrombocytopenia also may result from immunosuppression, especially with sirolimus, so the platelet count should be monitored frequently (see VIII.C.).

G.2. Hepatic toxicity

Several immunosuppressive agents cause or contribute to hepatic toxicity. Therefore, levels of alanine aminotransferase, aspartate aminotransferase, alkaline phosphatase, and bilirubin are measured at posttransplant months 1, 3, 6, and 12, and then annually thereafter (see VIII.C.).

G.3. Cardiovascular disease

G.3.a. Screening for cardiovascular disease

For patients with known ischemic heart disease, the patient's cardiologist may recommend periodic screening, usually with a noninvasive stress test. For asymptomatic patients without known ischemic heart disease, the role of periodic screening is unknown.

Similarly, the utility of screening patients for carotid artery disease via ultrasound is unclear. The US Preventative Services Task Force found insufficient evidence to recommend for or against screening asymptomatic individuals in the general population for carotid artery stenosis.[29] However, a recommendation for screening of high-risk patients could be made based on other grounds, provided high quality vascular surgical care is available. The US Preventative Services Task Force recommended against screening asymptomatic individuals in the general population for peripheral vascular disease.[30]

G.3.b. Prevention of cardiovascular disease

G.3.b.(1) Smoking cessation

Cigarette smoking is a major risk factor for cardiovascular disease (CVD) after transplantation. Patients should be periodically questioned about their smoking habits and strongly encouraged to abstain from cigarette smoking. Whenever possible, individuals who continue to smoke should be referred to a smoking cessation program with expertise in managing nicotine replacement therapies.

G.3.b.(2) Aspirin prophylaxis

In the general population, aspirin has been shown to reduce cardiovascular disease (CVD) events and overall mortality in patients with a history of myocardial infarction, stroke, transient ischemic attack, or other evidence of CVD.[31] A low dose of aspirin (75 mg) appears to be as effective as higher doses.[31,32] Aspirin also may be effective prophylactic therapy in patients without known CVD,[31] although the evidence is less convincing.[33] The American Diabetes Association recommends the use of aspirin in patients with type I or type II diabetes and additional risk factors for CVD.[34] Since the incidence of CVD is very high after transplantation, aspirin prophylaxis also may be beneficial in kidney transplant recipients with CVD as well as high-risk patients without CVD.

G.3.b.(3) Treatment of dyslipidemias

Approximately 80% of adult kidney transplant recipients have total cholesterol levels greater than 200 mg/dL, and 90% have low-density lipoprotein (LDL) cholesterol levels greater than 100 mg/dL. As most also have other risk factors for cardiovascular disease (CVD), the majority of adult kidney transplant recipients require treatment for their elevated LDL-cholesterol levels. Treatment should generally include both dietary modification and an HMG-CoA reductase inhibitor. The dose of most HMG-CoA inhibitors should be reduced in patients who are also receiving a calcineurin inhibitor.

G.3.b.(4) Posttransplant hypertension

Hypertension occurs in 50% to 80% of kidney transplant recipients.[1] Blood pressure should be treated to a target of less than 130 mm Hg systolic and less than 85 mm Hg diastolic. A lower blood pressure target may be even more desirable, if it can be achieved without causing adverse effects.[1]

No antihypertensive agent is absolutely contraindicated after transplantation. However, a number of special considerations should guide agent choice. Difficult-to-control hypertension should prompt screening for and/or correction of allograft vascular stenosis (<5% in most series). In some cases, native kidney nephrectomy may be necessary as a "last resort" measure for controlling blood pressure. The following table summarizes advantages ("Pros") and disadvantages ("Cons") of using various antihypertensive agents in renal transplant recipients:

Pros and Cons of Antihypertensive Agents		
Agent	**Pros**	**Cons**
Angiotensin-converting enzyme (ACE) inhibitors or receptor blockers	Cardioprotective Renoprotective ↓Proteinuria, ↓Hgb	↑Creatinine ↑Potassium ↓Hgb
Beta-blockers	Cardioprotective	Dyslipidemias
Dihydropyridine calcium antagonists	↑GFR	↑Mortality (?)
Non-dihydropyridine calcium antagonists	↑GFR, ↑CsA levels	↑CsA levels
Diuretics	↓Edema	↓GFR, dyslipidemias
Vasodilators	Potency	Edema

Abbreviations: Hgb, hemoglobin; GFR, glomerular filtration rate; CsA, cyclosporine.

G.4. Posttransplant diabetes

Diabetes in patients without preexisting diabetes (at transplantation) occurs in about 15% of transplant recipients during the first year.[35] Risk factors for posttransplant diabetes include older age, African American or Hispanic ethnicity, obesity, and a family history of diabetes. Corticosteroids, cyclosporine, and especially tacrolimus increase the risk of posttransplant diabetes. Altering the dose or discontinuing one of these immunosuppressive agents may cause remission. In any case, fasting blood glucose levels should be obtained at regular intervals after transplantation to screen for hyperglycemia and posttransplant diabetes (see VIII.C.).

G.5. Metabolic bone disease

G.5.a. Osteoporosis

Osteoporosis (bone mineral density >2.5 standard deviations below the young adult mean value t-score) may occur in as many as 60% of transplant recipients during the first 18 months posttransplant.[1] Although the incidence of osteoporosis in patients treated with steroid-reduction protocols remains unclear, it is probably lower but not zero. Mineral density of the lumbar spine and hip bone should generally be measured by dual x-ray absorptiometry before transplantation, 6 months after transplantation, and then every 12 months, if abnormal.[1] Effective treatment for corticosteroid-induced bone loss is available, but few randomized controlled trials have examined strategies for preventing osteoporosis in transplant recipients.[36,37]

G.5.b. Secondary hyperparathyroidism

Hypercalcemia occurs in 10% to 20% of transplant recipients during the first year;[1] therefore, patients should undergo periodic measurement of serum calcium levels posttransplant (see VIII.C.). The incidence of secondary hyperparathyroidism is poorly defined, but it is probably decreasing with improved pretransplant management of calcium and phosphorus. Nevertheless, some transplant recipients may require parathyroidectomy to control progressive bone demineralization, symptomatic hypercalcemia, or asymptomatic moderate hypercalcemia.[38]

G.6. Electrolyte abnormalities

G.6.a. Hypophosphatemia

Hypophosphatemia is extremely common early after transplantation.[1] The incidence of and severity of hypophosphatemia may be less in recipients on corticosteroid-free immunosuppressive protocols.[39] Severe hypophosphatemia may lead to muscle weakness and osteomalacia. Although few randomized trials have demonstrated the benefits of phosphorus replacement,[40] treatment of severe (and possibly mild) hypophosphatemia is probably warranted.

G.6.b. Hypomagnesemia

Hypomagnesemia may occur in as many as 25% of calcineurin inhibitor-treated, transplant recipients.[41,42] Hypomagnesemia may have a number of adverse consequences, including dyslipidemia and exacerbation of calcineurin inhibitor-related toxicity. Treatment with oral replacement of magnesium is safe and effective.

G.6.c. Hyperkalemia and metabolic acidosis

Hyperkalemia is particularly common in transplant recipients, especially those treated with calcineurin inhibitors. It is often associated with a mild, hyperchloremic metabolic acidosis. Since hyperkalemia is potentially life threatening, monitoring of serum potassium levels is warranted.

G.7. Nutritional complications

G.7.a. Hypoalbuminemia

Low serum albumin levels are common after transplantation. Approximately 10% of transplant recipients have hypoalbuminemia at 1 year, and the prevalence increases to greater than 20% by 10 years.[43] Hypoalbuminemia is associated with increased mortality after kidney transplantation.[43] Although some hypoalbuminemia may be due to malnutrition, hypoalbuminemia is also a reverse acute-phase reactant. Therefore, transplant recipients with cardiovascular disease or other complications that increase the risk of mortality may be more likely to have hypoalbuminemia. It follows that screening for hypoalbuminemia is indicated in transplant recipients.[1]

G.7.b. Obesity

Obesity is common after kidney transplantation. Although corticosteroids are suspected of being a major cause of this obesity, some posttransplant weight gain may reflect improved appetite and nutrition in patients who had lost weight prior to transplantation. Obesity may have an adverse effect on the risk of cardiovascular disease and is also associated with other complications.[44] Therefore, patients should be monitored for weight gain, and obese patients should be offered dietary counseling. Exercise should also be encouraged, although the benefits of exercise may not include weight loss.

G.8. Posttransplant malignancies

Cancer is responsible for 9% to 12% of deaths in renal transplant recipients.[1] In fact, the incidence of cancer is increased among kidney transplant recipients compared to age- and gender-matched controls from the general population.[45] Cancers for which viral infections may play a role in the pathogenesis, including lymphomas, Kaposi's sarcoma, cervical carcinoma, hepatic cell carcinoma, and skin cancers, are particularly common in transplant recipients compared to controls. In contrast, some cancers (e.g., breast cancer, prostate cancer) do not appear to be more common in transplant recipients. The following table summarizes the types of malignancies encountered after kidney transplantation and their risk ratios:

Types and Risks of Malignancy after Kidney Transplantation[a]	
Type/Location of Malignancy[c]	Risk Ratio (95% C.I.)[b]
Central nervous system lymphoma (17)	>1000 (939- >10,000)[d]
Ureter (10)	250 (120-460)[d]
Kaposi's sarcoma (18)	85.7 (50.8-135.5)[d]
Vulva/vagina (40)	43.5 (30.1-58.0)[d]
Cervix—in situ (50)	13.51 (10.03-17.82)[d]
Non-Hodgkin's lymphoma (83)	7.40 (5.90-9.18)[d]
Bladder (54)	7.19 (5.40-9.39)[d]
Kidney (54)	6.90 (5.18-9.00)[d]
Liver (8)	5.67 (2.45-11.18)[d]
Esophagus (14)	5.04 (2.49-8.00)[d]
Cervix—invasive (15)	3.78 (2.11-6.23)[d]
Leukemia (27)	3.60 (2.37-5.23)[d]
Thyroid (11)	3.42 (1.71-6.13)[d]
Colon (50)	2.26 (1.68-2.98)[d]
Buccal cavity (30)	2.52 (1.70-3.60)[d]
Pancreas (13)	2.77 (1.47-4.73)[d]
Trachea, bronchus, lung (60)	2.10 (1.61-2.71)[d]
Uterus (11)	1.63 (0.81-2.92)
Rectum and anus (22)	1.43 (0.90-2.16)
Stomach (9)	1.39 (1.18-3.64)[d]
Breast (44)	1.00 (0.73-1.14)
Prostate (21)	0.66 (0.41-1.01)
Total (785)	3.50 (2.64-3.04)[d]

[a]Data are from the Australia and New Zealand Dialysis and Transplant Registry of cadaveric donor kidneys (n=8618) transplanted 1965-1997.[45] Not shown are malignancies with fewer than 8 cases.

[b]Values are observed-to-expected (compared to age-matched controls) with 95% confidence intervals.

[c]Numbers in parentheses indicate the number of tumors in transplant recipients.

[d]Failure of the confidence intervals to include zero indicates the risk difference is statistically significant.

G.8.a. Cancer screening tests

In general, methods of screening for cancer after transplantation are the same as those recommended for the general population. Women older than 40 years of age should have a mammogram every 2 years to screen for breast cancer.[46] Women 18 years or older, as well as girls younger than 18 years who are sexually active, should undergo annual pelvic examination with a Pap smear.[47-50] Men 50 years or older with at least a 10-year life expectancy should undergo digital rectal examination and determination of prostate-specific antigen (PSA) levels to screen for prostate cancer.[51] In addition, transplant recipients 50 years or older should undergo screening for colorectal cancer with annual fecal occult blood testing and flexible sigmoidoscopy or colonoscopy every 5 years.[52-55]

The very high incidence of skin cancer in transplant recipients warrants at least annual skin examination by a physician. Patients also should be instructed to perform monthly skin self-examinations (best done by a significant other), avoid sun exposure, and use protective clothing. Patients with a history of skin cancer should see a dermatologist at least annually.

G.8.b. Monitoring of viruses linked to cancer

Although many malignancies are likely caused by viruses, there are no proven effective, prophylactic antiviral measures. Monitoring of viruses may or may not be effective. In particular, there is insufficient evidence that measuring the Epstein-Barr virus (EBV) load in peripheral blood is an effective means of screening for posttransplant lymphoproliferative disease (PTLD).[1] Similarly, there are insufficient data to suggest that measuring EBV gene expression in tissue (e.g., the allograft) effectively screens for PTLD. Monitoring EBV serologies, EBV oropharyngeal shedding, and serum monoclonal immunoglobulins also are not helpful strategies for preventing PTLD.

G.9. Infectious complications

G.9.a. Cytomegalovirus (CMV)

The presence of latent CMV infection in the donor, the amount of immunosuppressive medication, and the prophylactic use of antiviral agents determine both the risk and severity of CMV infection in a transplant recipient. With the advent of effective antiviral agents, the incidence of CMV infection has declined substantially in recent years. Currently, all kidney transplant recipients receive intravenous ganciclovir immediately after transplantation, which is followed by oral acyclovir for a total of 12 weeks.[1]

G.9.b. Influenza

Influenza is a potentially fatal, preventable infection in kidney transplant recipients. It is at least as common, and probably more severe, in transplant recipients compared to individuals in the general population. Studies have shown that 50% to 100% of kidney transplant recipients mount an antibody response to vaccination.[1] Therefore, patients should receive annual influenza vaccinations between October and November. Health care workers who have contact with transplant patients also should be vaccinated to prevent transmission.

During outbreaks of influenza, transplant recipients should be monitored closely. Patients without prior vaccination should be considered for prophylaxis, especially if they are receiving high doses of immunosuppressive medications.[56] Oral therapy with a neuraminidase inhibitor should be started within 48 hours of the onset of symptoms.

G.9.c. *Streptococcus pneumoniae*

The incidence of pneumococcal infection after kidney transplantation is not well defined, but it is probably about 1% per year. Vaccination is safe and effective, although the antibody response may not be as strong or as durable as it is in the general population. Therefore, polyvalent pneumococcal vaccine (capsular polysaccharides) should be administered, probably as often as every 2 years.[1]

G.9.d. Tuberculosis

The incidence of tuberculosis in kidney transplant recipients is estimated to be about 1% in North America. The risk for tuberculosis is higher in individuals from areas of the world where the disease is endemic (e.g., Southeast Asia). Screening and prophylaxis for tuberculosis are part of the pretransplant evaluation. However, high-risk patients should probably be monitored closely for tuberculosis during the posttransplant period.

G.9.e. *Pneumocystis carinii* pneumonia

Before effective prophylaxis was available, the incidence of *Pneumocystis carinii* pneumonia was as high as 10%. Now, cases are rare and usually occur in patients not receiving prophylaxis. Prophylaxis with trimethoprim-sulfamethoxazole is used in most patients. Alternative treatment for patients who cannot tolerate trimethoprim-sulfamethoxazole is dapsone, pentamidine, or atovaquone. Prophylaxis should be used during periods of intensive immunosuppression (e.g., the first few weeks after transplantation) as well as during treatment for acute rejection. However, the optimal duration of prophylaxis is unknown.

G.9.f. Hepatitis B

The prevalence of hepatitis B virus (HBV) infection is probably about 2% in North America.[1] Hepatitis B is usually acquired prior to transplantation, and patients with adequate pretransplant screening for HBV do not require routine posttransplant screening. Patients who have not had HBV should be vaccinated prior to transplantation. HBsAg-positive patients are generally treated with lamivudine 100 mg per day, starting at the time of transplantation and continuing for at least 18 to 24 months.

G.9.g. Hepatitis C

Antibodies to hepatitis C virus (anti-HCV) have been reported in 10% to 40% of renal transplant recipients.[1] The majority of seropositive patients have circulating HCV RNA in their serum.[57] Infection with HCV may be associated with a higher risk of sepsis and death from liver disease. Although screening (and sometimes treatment) of hepatitis C is an important part of the pretransplant evaluation, routine posttransplant screening is probably not helpful.

G.9.h. Candidiasis

Oral thrush and *Candida* esophagitis are relatively common in patients treated with high doses of immunosuppressive medications. Therefore, prophylaxis with mycostatin troches, 4 times daily, is warranted during the first few weeks after transplantation and during treatment for rejection.

BERT KASISKE, MD

References

1. Kasiske BL, Vazquez MA, Harmon WE, Danovitch GM, Danovitch GM, Gaston RS, et al. Recommendations for the outpatient surveillance of renal transplant recipients. *J Am Soc Nephrol.* 2000;11(10):S1.

2. Ross EA, Wilkinson A, Hawkins R, Danovitch GM. The plasma creatinine concentration is not an accurate reflection of the glomerular filtration rate in stable renal transplant patients receiving cyclosporine. *Am J Kidney Dis.* 1987;10:113-117.

3. Tomlanovich S, Golbetz H, Perlroth M, Stinson E, Myers BD. Limitations of creatinine in quantifying the severity of cyclosporine-induced chronic nephropathy. *Am J Kidney Dis.* 1986;8:332-337.

4. Schuck O, Matl I, Nadvornikova H, Teplan V, Skibova J. Cyclosporine A treatment and evaluation of glomerular filtration rate in patients with a transplanted kidney. *Int J Clin Pharmacol Ther Toxicol.* 1992;30(6):195-201.

5. Brown SCW, O'Reilly PH. Iohexol clearance for the determination of glomerular filtration rate in clinical practice: evidence for a new gold standard. *J Urol.* 1991;146:675-679.

6. Gaspari F, Perico N, Matalone M, Signorini O, Azzollini N, Mister M, et al. Precision of plasma clearance of iohexol for estimation of GFR in patients with renal disease. *J Am Soc Nephrol.* 1998;9:310-313.

7. Rydström M, Tengström B, Cederquist I, Ahlmén J. Measurement of glomerular filtration rate by single-injection, single-sample techniques, using 51CR-EDTA or iohexol. *Scand J Urol Nephrol.* 1995;29:135-139.

8. Sterner G. Iohexol clearance for GFR-determination in renal failure — single or multiple plasma sampling? *Nephrol Dial Transplant.* 1996;11:521-525.

9. Lundqvist S, Hietala SO, Groth S, Sjodin JG. Evaluation of single sample clearance calculations of 902 patients. A comparison of multiple and single sample techniques. *Acta Radiol.* 1997;38(1):68-72.

10. Chowdhury TA, Dyer PH, Bartlett WA, Legge ES, Durbin SM, Barnett AH, et al. Glomerular filtration rate determination in diabetic patients using iohexol clearance—comparison of single and multiple plasma sampling methods. *Clin Chim Acta.* 1998;277(2):153-158.

11. Gaspari F, Guerini E, Perico N, Mosconi L, Ruggenenti P, Remuzzi G. Glomerular filtration rate determined from a single plasma sample after intravenous iohexol injection: Is it reliable? *J Am Soc Nephrol.* 1996;7:2689-2693.

12. Kannel WB, Stampfer MJ, Castelli WP, Verter J. The prognostic significance of proteinuria: the Framingham study. *Am Heart J.* 1984;108:1347-1352.

13. Bulpitt CJ, Beevers DG, Butler A, Coles EC, Hunt D, Munro-Faure AD, et al. The survival of treated hypertensive patients and their causes of death: a report from the DHSS hypertensive care computing project (DHCCP). *J Hypertension.* 1986;4:93-99.

14. Samuelsson O, Wilhelmsen L, Elmfeldt D, Pennert K, Wedel H, Wikstrand J, et al. Predictors of cardiovascular morbidity in treated hypertension: Results from the primary preventive trial in Goteborg, Sweden. *J Hypertension.* 1985;3:167-176.

15. Keane WF, Eknoyan G. Proteinuria, albuminuria, risk, assessment, detection, elimination (PARADE): a position paper of the National Kidney Foundation. *Am J Kidney Dis.* 1999;33(5):1004-1010.

16. Mahalati K, Belitsky P, Sketris I, West K, Panek R. Neoral monitoring by simplified sparse sampling area under the concentration-time curve: its relationship to acute rejection and cyclosporine nephrotoxicity early after kidney transplantation. *Transplantation.* 1999;68(1):55-62.

17. Marsh CL. Abbreviated pharmacokinetic profiles in area-under-the-curve monitoring of cyclosporine therapy in de novo renal transplant patients treated with Sandimmune or Neoral. Neoral study group. *Ther Drug Monit.* 1999;21(1):27-34.

18. Wacke R, Rohde B, Engel G, Kundt G, Hehl EM, Bast R, et al. Comparison of several approaches of therapeutic drug monitoring of cyclosporin A based on individual pharmacokinetics. *Eur J Clin Pharmacol.* 2000;56(1):43-48.

19. Mahalati K, Belitsky P, West K, Kiberd B, Fraser A, Sketris I, et al. Approaching the therapeutic window for cyclosporine in kidney transplantation: a prospective study. *J Am Soc Nephrol.* 2001;12(4):828-833.

20. Perner F, International Neoral Renal Transplantation Study Group. Cyclosporine microemulsion (Neoral) absorption profiling and sparse-sample predictors during the first 3 months after renal transplantation. *Am J Transplant.* 2002;2:148-156.

21. Holt DW, Armstrong VW, Griesmacher A, Morris RG, Napoli KL, Shaw LM. International Federation of Clinical Chemistry/International Association of Therapeutic Drug Monitoring and Clinical Toxicology working group on immunosuppressive drug monitoring. *Ther Drug Monit.* 2002;24(1):59-67.

22. Staatz C, Taylor P, Tett S. Low tacrolimus concentrations and increased risk of early acute rejection in adult renal transplantation. *Nephrol Dial Transplant.* 2001;16(9):1905-1909.

23. Macchi-Andanson M, Charpiat B, Jelliffe RW, Ducerf C, Fourcade N, Baulieux J. Failure of traditional trough levels to predict tacrolimus concentrations. *Ther Drug Monit.* 2001;23(2):129-133.

24. Hale MD, Nicholls AJ, Bullingham RE, Hene R, Hoitsma A, Squifflet JP, et al. The pharmacokinetic-pharmacodynamic relationship for mycophenolate mofetil in renal transplantation. *Clin Pharmacol Ther.* 1998;64(6):672-683.

25. Le Guellec C, Büchler M, Giraudeau B, Le Meur Y, Gakoué JE, Lebranchu Y, et al. Simultaneous estimation of cyclosporin and mycophenolic acid areas under the curve in stable renal transplant patients using a limited sampling strategy. *Eur J Clin Pharmacol.* 2002;57(11):805-811.

26. Willis C, Taylor PJ, Salm P, Tett SE, Pillans PI. Evaluation of limited sampling strategies for estimation of 12-hour mycophenolic acid area under the plasma concentration-time curve in adult renal transplant patients. *Ther Drug Monit.* 2000;22(5):549-554.

27. MacDonald A, Scarola J, Burke JT, Zimmerman JJ. Clinical pharmacokinetics and therapeutic drug monitoring of sirolimus. *Clin Ther.* 2000;22(suppl B):B101-B121.

28. Kahan BD, Napoli KL, Kelly PA, Podbielski J, Hussein I, Urbauer DL, et al. Therapeutic drug monitoring of sirolimus: correlations with efficacy and toxicity. *Clin Transplant.* 2000;14(2):97-109.

29. U.S. Preventive Services Task Force. Screening for asymptomatic carotid artery stenosis. *Guide to Clinical Preventive Services.* 2nd ed. Baltimore, MD: Williams & Wilkins; 1996:53-61.

30. U.S. Preventive Services Task Force. Screening for peripheral arterial disease. *Guide to Clinical Preventive Services.* 2nd ed. Baltimore, MD: Williams & Wilkins; 1996:63-66.

31. Collaborative overview of randomised trials of antiplatelet therapy—I: Prevention of death, myocardial infarction, and stroke by prolonged antiplatelet therapy in various categories of patients. Antiplatelet Trialists' Collaboration. *BMJ.* 1994;308(6921):81-106.

32. Johnson ES, Lanes SF, Wentworth CE, Satterfield MH, Abebe BL, Dicker LW. A metaregression analysis of the dose-response effect of aspirin on stroke. *Arch Intern Med.* 1999;159(11):1248-1253.

33. U.S. Preventive Services Task Force. Aspirin prophylaxis for the primary prevention of myocardial infarction. In: Di Guiseppi C, Atkins D, Woolf S, eds. *Guide to Clinical Preventive Services.* 2nd ed. Baltimore, MD: Williams & Wilkins; 1996:845-852.

34. Aspirin therapy in diabetes. American Diabetes Association. *Diabetes Care.* 1997;20(11):1772-1773.

35. Kasiske BL, Snyder JJ, Gilbertson D, Matas AJ. Diabetes mellitus after kidney transplantation in the United States. *Am J Transplant.* 2003;3(2):178-185.

36. Cueto-Manzano AM, Konel S, Freemont AJ, Adams JE, Mawer B, Gokal R, et al. Effect of 1,25-dihydroxy vitamin D3 and calcium carbonate on bone loss associated with long-term renal transplantation. *Am J Kidney Dis.* 2000;35(2):227-236.

37. Fan SL, Almond MK, Ball E, Evans K, Cunningham J. Pamidronate therapy as prevention of bone loss following renal transplantation. *Kidney Int.* 2000;57(2):684-690.

38. Schmid T, Muller P, Spelsberg F. Parathyroidectomy after renal transplantation: a retrospective analysis of long-term outcome. *Nephrol Dial Transplant.* 1997;12(11):2393-2396.

39. Higgins RM, Richardson AJ, Endre ZH, Frostick SP, Morris PJ. Hypophosphataemia after renal transplantation: relationship to immunosuppressive drug therapy and effects on muscle detected by 31P nuclear magnetic resonance spectroscopy. *Nephrol Dial Transplant.* 1990;5(1):62-68.

40. Ambuhl PM, Meier D, Wolf B, Dydak U, Boesiger P, Binswanger U. Metabolic aspects of phosphate replacement therapy for hypophosphatemia after renal transplantation: impact on muscular phosphate content, mineral metabolism, and acid/base homeostasis. *Am J Kidney Dis.* 1999;34(5):875-883.

41. Scoble JE, Freestone A, Varghese Z, Fernando ON, Sweny P, Moorhead JF. Cyclosporin-induced renal magnesium leak in renal transplant patients. *Nephrol Dial Transplant.* 1990;5(9):812-815.

42. Vannini SD, Mazzola BL, Rodoni L, Truttmann AC, Wermuth B, Bianchetti MG, et al. Permanently reduced plasma ionized magnesium among renal transplant recipients on cyclosporine. *Transpl Int.* 1999;12(4):244-249.

43. Guijarro C, Massy ZA, Ma JZ, Wiederkehr M, Kasiske BL. Serum albumin and mortality after renal transplantation. *Am J Kidney Dis*. 1996;27(1):117-123.

44. Saad MF, Knowler WC, Pettitt DJ, Nelson RG, Mott DM, Bennett PH. The natural history of impaired glucose tolerance in the Pima Indians. *N Engl J Med*. 1988;319(23):1500-1506.

45. Sheil AGR. Cancer Report. In: Disney APS, ed. Australia and New Zealand Dialysis and Transplant Registry 1997. Adelaide, South Australia: ANZDATA Registry, 1998:138-146.

46. National Cancer Institute. *Screening for Breast Cancer*. 1998. National Institutes of Health.

47. ter Haar-van Eck SA, Rischen-Vos J, Chadha-Ajwani S, Huikeshoven FJM. The incidence of cervical intraepithelial neoplasia among women with renal transplant in relation to cyclosporine. *Br J Obstet Gynaecol*. 1995;102:58-61.

48. National Cancer Institute. *Screening for Cervical Cancer*. 1996. National Institutes of Health.

49. ACOG Committee. Recommendations on frequency of Pap test screening. ACOG Committee Opinion 1995;152:1.

50. U.S. Preventive Services Task Force. Screening for cervical cancer. In: Di Guiseppi C, Atkins D, Woolf S, eds. *Guide to Clinical Preventive Services*. 2nd ed. Baltimore, MD: Williams & Wilkins; 1996:105-117.

51. American College of Physicians. Screening for prostate cancer. *Ann Intern Med*. 1997;126:480-484.

52. U.S.Preventive Services Task Force. Screening for colorectal cancer. In: Di Guiseppi C, Atkins D, Woolf S, eds. *Guide to Clinical Preventive Services*. 2nd ed. Baltimore, MD: Williams & Wilkins; 1996:89-103.

53. Byers T, Levin B, Rothenberger D, Dodd GD, Smith RA. American Cancer Society guidelines for screening and surveillance for early detection of colorectal polyps and cancer: update 1997. *CA Cancer J Clin*. 1998;47:154-160.

54. National Cancer Institute. *Screening for Colorectal Cancer*. 1998. National Institutes of Health.

55. Winawer SJ, Fletcher RH, Miller L, Godlee F, Stolar MH, Mulrow CD, et al. Colorectal cancer screening: clinical guidelines and rationale. *Gastroenterology.* 1997;112:594-642.

56. Prevention and control of influenza: recommendations of the Advisory Committee on Immunization Practices (ACIP). *MMWR Morb Mortal Wkly Rep.* 2000;49(RR-3):1-38.

57. Roth D, Zucker K, Cirocco R, DeMattos A, Burke GW, Nery J, et al. The impact of hepatitis C virus infection on renal allograft recipients. *Kidney Int.* 1994;45(1):238-244.

IX. Pediatric Kidney Transplantation

Compared to chronic dialysis, kidney transplantation offers children greater potential for growth and development and achievement of a normal lifestyle. The field has undergone remarkable advances in the last 2 decades with the introduction of new medications to treat rejection. The 1-year patient survival rates have ranged from 95% to 98% since the early 1980s. In addition, 1-year graft survival rates have increased from 85% in the early 1980s to 90% at present. The major reasons for the increase in graft survival include earlier referral of children with end-stage kidney disease, improved surgical and preservation techniques, better immunosuppressive regimens, and greater experience of the transplant care team.

A. Program Description

A.1. Program history

Pediatric kidney transplantation has been performed at the University of Minnesota/Fairview-University Medical Center (F-UMC) since 1963. We have performed more than 800 transplants in children and adolescents ranging in age from 6 months to 19 years.[1] A major strength of this program has been kidney transplantation in infants and small children; more than a third of the infant transplants performed nationwide have been performed here.[2,3]

Several transplant firsts important to pediatric kidney transplantation have taken place at F-UMC. We pioneered the use of adult kidneys for kidney transplantation in infants and small children. Our center was the first to show that it is possible to achieve patient and graft survival rates for children younger than 4 years that do not differ from those for adults or children aged 5 to 17 years. Successful strategies for kidney transplantation in children with systemic oxalosis were first developed here. We were the first to report neurologic improvement in infants after kidney transplantation. We also were the first to report the recurrence of steroid-resistant nephrotic syndrome in the transplanted kidney. In addition, we showed that trough cyclosporine concentrations of less than 100 ng/mL during the first year posttransplant were a risk factor for acute and chronic rejection. The University of Minnesota/Fairview-University Medical Center (F-UMC) continues to pursue improvements in graft survival rates, posttransplant complication rates, and quality of life in children.

A.2. Contact information

The members of the pediatric transplantation team and their phone numbers are as follows:

Transplant surgeons

David L. Dunn, MD, PhD	612.626.1999
Rainer W. Gruessner, MD	612.625.1485
Abhinav Humar, MD	612.624.0688
Raja Kandaswamy, MD	612.625.7997
Arthur J. Matas, MD, PhD	612.625.6460
John S. Najarian, MD, PhD	612.625.8444
William D. Payne, MD	612.625.5151
David Sutherland, MD, PhD	612.625.7600

Pediatric nephrologists

Michael Bendel-Stenzel, MD	612.626.2922
Blanche Chavers, MD	612.626.2922
Elizabeth Ingulli, MD	612.626.2922
Clifford Kashtan, MD	612.626.2922
Michael Mauer, MD	612.626.2922
Thomas Nevins, MD	612.626.2922

Transplant coordinators

Marie Cook, RN, CPNP, MPH, CCTC	612.625.4166
Marci Knaak, RN	612.625.8666

Social worker

Kathy Weck, MSW	612.273.4936

Financial representatives

A-G	James Roscoe	612.273.6742
H & M	Susan Weisz	612.273.3110
I-L	John Diamond	612.273.6879
N-V	Beth Van der Loop	612.273.6239
W-Z	Kenneth Reid	612.273.6795

B. Pretransplant Issues

B.1. Indications for transplantation

Kidney transplantation is indicated for patients with chronic kidney failure. The list of kidney diseases once thought to be unsuitable for transplantation has shortened as our experience with transplantation has increased. Generally, any child who requires renal replacement therapy is a candidate for kidney transplantation.

The causes of end-stage kidney disease in childhood are varied. According to the United States Renal Data System registry, the most common single cause in children is primary glomerulonephritis (GN) (29.8% of all reported cases).[4] Diseases encompassed in the primary GN category include focal glomerulosclerosis, membranous nephropathy, membranoproliferative GN, IgA nephropathy, rapidly progressive GN, Goodpasture's syndrome, and other unspecified GN.

Cystic/hereditary/congenital diseases are the second largest category of diseases that results in childhood end-stage kidney disease (26% of reported cases). Diseases in this category include polycystic kidney disease, medullary cystic disease, Alport's syndrome, cystinosis, oxalosis, congenital nephrotic syndrome, congenital obstructive uropathy, hypoplasia/dysplasia, and prune belly syndrome.

The four most common diseases are unspecified GN (10.3%), focal glomerulosclerosis (10.2%), dysplasia/hypoplasia (8.9%), and congenital obstructive uropathy (6.7%). Early in life, the most common causes of end-stage kidney disease are congenital structural lesions such as obstruction; GN is the most common cause later in life. Interstitial nephritis and collagen-vascular disease/vasculitis each account for about 9% of all reported cases of kidney failure in childhood. Hypertension and renal artery stenosis or occlusion account for approximately 5% of cases. The five most common causes of end-stage kidney disease in children transplanted at our center over the past 10 years have been obstructive uropathy, GN, congenital anomalies, congenital nephrotic syndrome, and focal segmental glomerulosclerosis.

In 1998, the Pediatric Committee of the American Society of Transplantation published a position paper in *Pediatric Transplantation* on indications for and special considerations regarding pediatric kidney transplantation.[5] Their recommended indications for kidney transplantation include:

- End-stage kidney disease unresponsiveness to medical management.
- Progressive growth failure and failure to thrive.
- Progressive renal osteodystrophy.
- Developmental delay.

B.1.a. Malnutrition, growth failure, and failure to thrive

Marked metabolic and biochemical changes develop in children once the kidney loses its ability to function normally. Malnutrition is related to the nausea and lack of appetite these children develop as the kidney disease progresses. This anorexia affects their daily calorie and vitamin intake. Some children develop gastroesophageal reflux and gastric dysmotility, which contribute to feeding difficulties. In addition, consumed calories may not be used efficiently.

Nutrition must be maximized in children with kidney failure, especially infants. Both weight gain and adequacy of nutrition must be appropriately addressed. Generally, the less debilitated the child is at the time of transplantation, the lower the morbidity and mortality following the procedure. Therefore, every attempt should be made to optimize nutrition and growth prior to proceeding to transplantation. Hypercaloric formulas (30-60 kcal/ounce) supplemented with protein, glucose polymers, and/or medium chain triglycerides are often required. These formulas are often given via a nasogastric, nasojejunal, or gastrostomy feeding tube. In addition, the child should be placed on a kidney failure diet, which involves reduced daily phosphorus intake, the use of phosphate binders, vitamin D supplementation, correction of acidosis, and in some patients, sodium chloride (salt) supplementation. Subcutaneously or intravenously administered recombinant human erythropoietin should be used to manage a low red blood cell count (anemia) associated with chronic renal disease.

The accumulation of acid in the body (acidosis) is common and, when present, interferes with the child's ability to grow. This is because the body uses buffers from bone (bone salts, calcium carbonate) to counteract this build-up of acid, and the child's growth suffers as a consequence. Causes of acidosis include the kidney's inability to excrete normal amounts of body acid (titratable acid) into the urine and the loss of buffer (bicarbonate) into the urine in some patients. The acidosis may stabilize, partially due to the tremendous buffering capacity of bone. Infants are most susceptible to growth failure. If the child shows no response to implementation of the above-described measures, recombinant human growth hormone can be administered in an attempt to accelerate growth. A potential long-term effect of buffering by bone is metabolic bone disease (see IX.B.1.b.).

B.1.b. Renal osteodystrophy (metabolic bone disease)

Renal osteodystrophy, resulting from secondary hyperparathyroidism, is a major contributor to growth failure. As kidney function worsens, there is a transient rise in the body's serum phosphate concentration accompanied by a decrease in ionized serum calcium. This stimulates an increase in parathyroid hormone, which increases the serum calcium level and decreases phosphate reabsorption. Kidney failure also leads to the reduced production of vitamin D, which decreases calcium absorption from the gut and serum calcium levels. Bone mineralization also may be abnormal in children with kidney failure. Collectively, these factors lead to skeletal abnormalities. Renal osteodystrophy is most pronounced in areas of rapid growth, such as the bones of the upper arm, knees, wrist, and clavicle. Metabolic bone disease may be accompanied by bone pain and rarely, fractures.

B.1.c. Developmental delay and central nervous system dysfunction

Many children with end-stage kidney disease will have retarded psychomotor development, especially those who develop kidney failure within the first year of life. The cause of this developmental delay is multifactorial and includes prolonged illness, frequent hospitalizations, prior surgery, anemia, malnutrition, and progressive uremia. Although many of these children are able to talk and interact socially with adults, they display muscle weakness, hypotonia, and difficulty walking and experience bone pain from metabolic bone disease. Infants demonstrate a delay in reaching developmental milestones. School-age children exhibit poor school attendance and reduced performance compared to healthy peers.

Infants may display even more profound central nervous system (CNS) abnormalities including lack of/insufficient growth in head size, seizures, and involuntary body movement (dyskinesia). In such cases, a formal neurological evaluation is required. A landmark paper published from our center by Rotundo et al. in 1982 showed that infants with chronic kidney failure had increased susceptibility to progressive encephalopathy.[6] This study suggested that the duration and degree of uremia should be minimized in infants and that early transplantation might be required to protect or stabilize the developing brain in these infants.

For children with severe, fixed, global CNS dysfunction whose parents have requested transplantation, we recommend that these issues be resolved at the level of the hospital's bioethics committee. This assures that the decision-making process reflects a broader constituency than that of an individual physician.

B.2. Biochemical abnormalities

As kidney function deteriorates, biochemical abnormalities develop. Laboratory evidence of this may include high serum concentrations of potassium, blood urea nitrogen (BUN), creatinine, phosphorus, and parathyroid hormone as well as low serum concentrations of bicarbonate, calcium, and sodium.

B.3. Contraindications to transplantation

Few absolute contraindications to kidney transplantation in children exist. The 1998 position paper by the Pediatric Committee of the American Society of Transplantation[5] addresses this issue. Contraindications to kidney transplantation in children include:

- Active malignancy or less than 12 months posttreatment for malignancy.
- Human immunodeficiency virus (HIV) infection.
- Positive current T-cell cross-match.
- History of active noncompliance with medical management.

The time to wait until transplantation following treatment of a malignancy is controversial. Many centers recommend waiting 2 years from the completion of treatment. Other centers have a minimum wait time of 1 year from completion of treatment for a malignancy.

At our center, we do not consider chronic active hepatitis B or C infection to be a contraindication to kidney transplantation. However, transplantation in these patients may be associated with an increased long-term risk of liver cirrhosis and failure as well as liver cancer (hepatocellular carcinoma).

Atresia or thrombosis of the inferior vena cava or aorta is not an absolute contraindication to kidney transplantation. However, prior review and planning by the transplant surgeon is required, as such transplantation is extremely difficult and may be unsuccessful.

A relative contraindication to transplantation would be lack of adequate home supervision or family support for long-term management of the transplant recipient. Substance abuse in the older pediatric patient is a contraindication to transplantation. Enrollment in a chemical dependency program and a minimum of 6 months of abstinence would be required before such patients would be considered for transplantation. Respirator-dependent patients or patients with severe multiorgan failure that precludes a combined transplant with a kidney are also unlikely transplant candidates.

B.4. Transplant timing

The timing of pediatric kidney transplantation is controversial. Age and size must be taken into consideration once it has been decided that the patient is a transplant candidate. Our approach at the University of Minnesota/Fairview-University Medical Center (F-UMC) is based on two premises: a) the outcome of transplantation with living donors is better than that with cadaveric donors and b) infants and small children with end-stage kidney failure do not grow and develop normally.

We believe that transplantation is a more effective treatment for infants and small children with kidney failure than chronic dialysis. Transplant centers vary regarding their minimum age and size requirements. Many centers use 12 to 24 months of age and a body weight of 10 kilograms as minimum requirements. Some centers, including ours, will transplant infants as young as 6 months of age, but they must weigh 6 to 10 kilograms.

B.5. Pretransplant nephrectomy

An important decision that must be made at the time of the child's evaluation is whether nephrectomy is required and if so, when it should be performed (i.e., before or at the time of transplantation). Indications for bilateral nephrectomy include children with malignant hypertension resistant to medical management, vesicoureteral reflux, and recurrent pyelonephritis. Avoidance of native nephrectomy in children with the former will result in many patients requiring life-long treatment with antihypertensive medication.

Nephroureterectomy may be performed either pretransplant (>20 kg body weight) or at the time of transplantation (<20 kg body weight). Because our approach in children weighing less than 20 kilograms is to transplant through a midline incision, a bilateral nephrectomy is usually performed in these patients at the time of transplantation, provided there are no contraindications. For older children who undergo transplantation via an extraperitoneal approach, the nephrectomy is done pretransplant.

Children with congenital or infantile nephrotic syndrome, hyper-coagulability due to the nephrotic state, or recurrent pyelonephritis will require nephrectomies performed at least 6 weeks prior to transplantation. Pretransplant nephrectomies are also performed in children with respiratory compromise or feeding difficulties related to large polycystic kidneys. The 6-week interval between pretransplant nephrectomy and kidney transplantation allows for postoperative and nutritional recovery as well as resolution of the hypercoagulable state (in patients with this complication of nephrotic syndrome). The bilateral posterior or loin incision approach is safer than the midline approach (lower incidence of ileus, fewer postoperative pulmonary complications), but it is unsuitable for ureterectomy or removal of very large kidneys.

C. Diseases Treatable by Kidney Transplantation That Require Special Attention

A host of diseases are potentially treatable by kidney transplantation. Several diseases leading to end-stage kidney disease in children pose special challenges in the preparation for transplantation.

C.1. Nephrotic syndrome

Children with nephrotic syndromes, such as congenital nephrotic syndrome, diffuse mesangial sclerosis, and focal segmental glomerulosclerosis, require pretransplant bilateral nephrectomy. This allows time for the resolution of body edema, facilitates aggressive nutritional therapy, and decreases the risk of infection, hyperlipidemia, and/or a hypercoagulable state, thus, diminishes the risk of posttransplant graft thrombosis. Dialysis is usually required for a minimum of 6 weeks after bilateral nephrectomy.

C.2. Diffuse mesangial sclerosis

Approximately 35% of patients with diffuse mesangial sclerosis (DMS) have a constellation of findings consistent with Drash syndrome, which may include Wilms' tumor, male pseudohermaphroditism (ambiguous genitalia), and gonadal dysgenesis. These children require chromosome karyotyping, genetic screening for the germline mutation in the Wilms' tumor suppressor gene, and bilateral gonadectomy. They should also undergo (serial) renal ultrasound examinations every 3 months, from the time of diagnosis until the time of transplantation, when bilateral nephrectomy should be performed. Children with DMS and nephrotic syndrome require pretransplant nephrectomy.

C.3. Obstructive uropathy and urologic abnormalities

Obstruction due to posterior urethral valves is the most common obstructive lesion in boys. Children with such urologic abnormalities require careful pretransplant evaluation of the bladder storage capacity, competency of the bladder neck, and patency of the urethra, as bladder dysfunction is common in patients with obstructive uropathy.[7] Manifestations of these abnormalities include bladder distention, dribbling, and poor urinary stream.

Urologic evaluation should include a renal ultrasound examination and a voiding cystourethogram. Often cystometrics or urodynamic evaluation is required to detect abnormalities in voiding patterns. Antispasmodic medication and/or intermittent catheterization may be required to minimize the transmission of high pressures to the renal pelvis; high pressures can impair drainage of the upper collecting system, resulting in reflux and/or diminished allograft function posttransplant.

The primary surgical treatment for posterior urethral valves is resection of the valves. The urologist and transplant surgeon usually determine surgical treatments. Surgical procedures, including reconstruction of the urethral sphincter or construction of an appendiceal stoma (Mitrofanoff procedure), should be performed pretransplant. In addition, pyelostomies and ureterostomies should be taken down prior to transplantation. Bladders not used for extended periods because of urinary diversion may have small capacities and poor function. However, in many of these cases, urinary continence can be achieved within a few months following successful undiversion or transplantation; augmentation of the bladder with ureter or gastrointestinal mucosa may not even be required. The unused bladder should be used once bladder outlet obstruction has been corrected.[7]

C.4. Oxalosis

Primary hyperoxaluria type I is an autosomal recessive inborn error of metabolism involving a deficiency in the hepatic peroxisomal enzyme alanine: glyoxylate aminotransferase. Children with oxalosis or primary hyperoxaluria type I overproduce oxalate and develop nephrocalcinosis, recurrent kidney stones (urolithiasis), and end-stage kidney disease. Since the excretion of oxalate is primarily via the kidney, significant quantities of oxalate are deposited in tissues of the skeletal and cardiovascular systems once the glomerular filtration rate (GFR) decreases to less than 40 mL/min.

Medical treatment of these patients includes high fluid intake, to maximize the urinary flow rate; thiazide diuretics, to reduce the rate of urinary calcium excretion; phosphorus and magnesium supplementation, to enhance oxalate solubility; and pyridoxine therapy, to decrease the amount of the oxalate precursor glyoxylate. Prior to transplantation, 6-times per week hemodialysis and nighttime peritoneal dialysis treatment are recommended to decrease total body oxalate stores and deposition. Combined liver/kidney transplantation is recommended for patients with severe oxalosis.

C.5. Autosomal recessive polycystic kidney disease (ARPKD)

Single or bilateral nephrectomy may be required in infants with autosomal recessive polycystic kidney disease (ARPKD) and uncontrollable hypertension or respiratory compromise due to nephromegaly. This disease is often associated with congenital hepatic fibrosis, which frequently leads to portal hypertension. Therefore, these patients need to be monitored for evidence of variceal bleeding, which is more common after the first decade of life. Because patients with ARPKD may require future portal vein shunting, careful planning with the pediatric surgeon is essential prior to any scheduled abdominal surgery.[8]

D. Pretransplant Evaluation and Management

D.1. Goals of the pretransplant evaluation

Ideally, children are referred for transplant evaluation before they reach end-stage kidney disease; however, this is often not the case. Early evaluation allows time to correct various problems (e.g., bladder outlet obstruction, bone deformities). It affords more time for assessing/understanding family dynamics and for providing patient and family education.

Once a child has been diagnosed with a disorder that only kidney transplantation can correct, the patient and family undergo extensive evaluation by the transplant team.[9] Most centers require that the patient travel to the center for this evaluation; however, this assessment can also be conducted on an outpatient basis. Purposes of the pretransplant evaluation include the following:

- To confirm or to establish a diagnosis through review of records and biopsy material.
- To assess the complications of end-stage renal disease.
- To assess anatomic suitability for transplantation and potential complicating anomalies (e.g., presence of an atretic inferior vena cava).
- To assess the psychosocial status of the child and family and anticipate support needs.
- To educate the patient and family about kidney transplantation.

Components of this evaluation include a complete patient history and physical examination, laboratory and other clinical tests/studies, consultations with various healthcare professionals, psychological evaluation, and patient and family education.

D.2. Components of the pretransplant evaluation

D.2.a. Patient history and physical examination

Table 9 outlines steps involved in our standard evaluation. At our institution, we use an evaluation checklist to help guide the evaluation and ensure appropriate completion. The evaluation begins with a complete history and physical examination. Growth data are documented, and the patient is screened for underlying cardiovascular abnormalities. Blood pressure control is also evaluated and, if necessary, measures are recommended to achieve adequate control before transplantation.

The patient is also screened for any type of infection. Potential foci of infection include the sinuses, urinary tract, ears, chest, peritoneal or hemodialysis catheter site, and peritoneum. Active peritonitis, as well as peritonitis that persists despite antibiotic treatment, are considered relative contraindications to transplantation. Most centers require that the patient be free of peritonitis for at least 4 weeks prior to transplantation. Dental caries should be treated to reduce the risk of a posttransplant dental abscess. A history of prior blood clotting or hypercoagulability, either in the patient or family members, also should be sought.

D.2.b. Laboratory tests

The following laboratory tests are included in the pediatric pretransplant evaluation:

- Complete blood count (CBC) with platelets.
- Chemistry profile including electrolytes, blood urea nitrogen (BUN), creatinine (Cr), calcium, phosphorus, and intact parathyroid hormone concentrations.
- Complete liver function tests, including serum liver enzymes, bilirubin, albumin, cholesterol, and triglyceride concentrations.
- Coagulation profile including an international normalized ratio (INR) and partial prothrombin time (to screen for coagulation abnormalities).
- Viral serology tests, including those for hepatitis A, B, and C; cytomegalovirus (CMV); Epstein-Barr virus (EBV); varicella-zoster; measles, mumps, and rubella; and human immunodeficiency virus (HIV).
- Blood bank ABO blood group and human leukocyte antigen (HLA) typing, antileukocyte antibody screening, and immunoglobulin concentrations.

   • Urinalysis, urine culture, and 24-hour urinary protein
     determination.

D.2.c. Other tests

Whenever possible, the potential donor's immune status
regarding cytomegalovirus (CMV) and Epstein-Barr virus (EBV)
should be obtained. These studies are important as transmission
of one of these viruses from a donor to the recipient may occur
after transplantation. Other tests included in the pretransplant
evaluation are as follows:

   • Chest radiograph (x-ray).
   • 12-lead electrocardiogram (ECG).
   • Peritoneal fluid (cell count and differential, culture if
     patient is undergoing peritoneal dialysis).
   • Ultrasound Doppler study of the native kidneys (to
     assess blood flow to the inferior vena cava and to rule
     out thrombosis).
   • Voiding cystourethrogram (to evaluate for
     urethral patency, vesicoureteral reflux, and residual
     urine volume).
   • Bone age.
   • Pap smear for girls older than 15 years or
     postmenarche.
   • Homocysteine levels, as well as a coagulation
     evaluation, for patients undergoing chronic dialysis or
     with a history of clotting.
   • Placement of Mantoux test (containing 5 tuberculin
     units of purified protein derivative [PPD]) with controls
     for *Candida* and mumps (to rule out tuberculosis and
     evaluate for a false-negative reaction due to uremia-
     induced suppression of the immune response).

D.2.d. Immunizations

The child's immunization status needs to be defined prior to
transplantation. The patient should be screened, as described
above, and steps should be taken to prevent posttransplant
infectious complications. We recommend routine childhood
vaccinations against preventable diseases as well as immunization
against pathogens linked to increased morbidity in transplant
patients (e.g., hepatitis B, pneumococcus, varicella, influenza).
Every effort should be made to immunize the child prior to
transplantation, as pretransplant immunizations decrease the

likelihood of the immunocompromised patient acquiring a life-threatening infection posttransplantation.

Live viral vaccines, such as measles-mumps-rubella or varicella, should be given 12 weeks before transplantation, since earlier administration of immunosuppression increases the risk of significant infection for this patient group. In addition, both the child and family members should receive the inactivated polio vaccine if renal transplantation is anticipated within the next 6 months to avoid contact with the live attenuated poliovirus. The hepatitis B series should be completed pretransplant, whenever possible. The child should receive the dialysis formulation, which is a larger dose. An annual influenza A and B vaccine should be administered if the child is older than 6 months of age. Children younger than 12 years should receive the split virus vaccine. Children receiving the influenza vaccine for the first time will usually require a second dose.

The varicella zoster virus causes both a systemic primary infection and a latent infection in sensory ganglia. Infectious complications of varicella can be life threatening. The varicella vaccine (Varivax), which is a live-attenuated vaccine, was released in 1995. It is recommended that the vaccine be given at any time on or after the first birthday in susceptible children. Titers should be checked 1 month after administration, and if nondetectable, a second dose should be administered.

The varicella vaccine is still being studied in the US and is currently only approved for use in healthy children. Immuno-suppression is considered a contraindication to vaccine administration. However, the safety of this vaccine is currently being evaluated in kidney transplant patients. Available studies suggest that the varicella vaccine is safe and effective in children with end-stage kidney disease. Therefore, we recommend administering it prior to transplantation. Data on adverse events associated with immunization with live viral vaccines after transplantation are available from the National Vaccine Adverse Events Reporting System (VAERS).

D.2.e. Consultations

The commitment made to care for and transplant children with end-stage renal disease is both challenging and rewarding, but it requires the commitment of a multidisciplinary team. This team evaluates the child pretransplant and then meets on a weekly basis to plan ongoing treatment for the child. Team members include:

- Pediatric nephrologist.
- Surgeon.
- Urologist.
- Neurologist.
- Psychiatrist/Psychologist.
- Transplant/Dialysis nurses.
- Transplant nurse coordinator.
- Dietitian.
- Social worker.
- Financial representative.
- Pediatric dentist.

Consultation with other healthcare professionals may be arranged, if necessary; these individuals may include:

- Anesthesiologist.
- Pediatric intensivist.
- Pediatric cardiologist.
- Transplant pharmacist.
- Child family life specialist.
- Occupational, physical, and speech therapists.

D.2.f. Patient/family education

Education of the transplant recipient and his or her family members begins early and takes several forms:

D.2.f.(1) Information packet

Prior to the evaluation, an information packet is sent to the family. The following table summarizes aspects of kidney transplantation addressed in this packet:

INFORMATION PACKET FOR PEDIATRIC KIDNEY TRANSPLANTATION

Paying for your transplant.
- Who pays?
- How do you know if you can receive a transplant at our center?
- How do services, medicines, and equipment get paid for after surgery?
- Types of insurance.
- Paying for costs not covered by insurance.

How to discuss living donation with family members and friends.

Review of our pediatric transplant program and outcomes.

Before your transplant.
- Transplant work-up.
- How long the work-up takes.
- Where to stay during the work-up.
- How to arrange/prepare for dialysis while in Minneapolis.
- Tests to be performed.
- Blood typing, tissue typing, cross-match, and antibody levels.
- Blood transfusions.
- Radiologic studies.

How to get on the cadaver waiting list.

What to do when you get the call to come in for a cadaveric kidney.

When to let the doctor know if your child is sick or had a recent infection.

When to give your child nothing by mouth (NPO).

D.2.f.(2) Pretransplant class

Parents and the potential transplant recipient (when appropriate) also attend a pretransplant class and video presentation designed for patients and their families. The class is held on a weekly basis and is taught by a transplant coordinator. Each potential transplant recipient and/or guardian attends at least one class. The following topics are discussed during the class:

- What to expect during the transplant hospitalization.
- Transplant medications and side effects.
- Possible complications after transplantation.
- Posttransplant monitoring.

D.3. Pretransplant evaluation checklist

After the work-up has been completed, a detailed checklist must be filled out before the candidate can be scheduled for a living-donor transplant or placed on the cadaveric kidney waiting list. This multipurpose form allows the dates and results of laboratory tests and consultations to be compiled onto a single sheet. A pediatric nephrologist or the transplant nurse coordinator usually completes this checklist, which is intended to ensure a thorough pretransplant evaluation.

D.4. Psychological factors

Psychological and social support for the families of children undergoing kidney transplantation is critical. Many families are unprepared to deal with a chronically ill child and the associated burdens they will face. It is not uncommon for the parents to experience feelings of guilt, anger, depression, and loss of control. They need help learning how to cope. Parents also need to understand both the medical and nonmedical consequences of the transplant procedure.

At the transplant center, social service and psychological evaluations are conducted to help identify at-risk families that may require more formal psychiatric intervention. All families with a child awaiting transplantation need to be made aware of the risk of failure or their acceptance of a return to dialysis will be more difficult. This especially applies to children who have diseases with a high rate of recurrence in the allograft. For example, focal segmental glomerulosclerosis has been reported to recur in 40% of children with mesangial proliferation on biopsy and progression to end-stage kidney disease within 3 years of diagnosis. Recurrence in retransplants approaches 60% to 80% once the primary graft is lost to recurrence. Hemolytic uremic syndrome (HUS; microangiopathic hemolytic anemia, uremia, thrombocytopenia) is the most common cause of acute renal failure in childhood and typically occurs after a diarrheal prodromal illness. The risk of recurrence of HUS in the renal allograft ranges from 10% to 25%, but it is negligible in patients with a classic diarrheal prodrome.[10]

Some families require therapeutic intervention and continuous counseling to help manage the mental health problems that tend to plague families with children who are in renal failure. Patients and families need to know that the duration of hospitalization after transplantation may be as brief as 5 to 7 days or quite prolonged, if complications ensue. For recipients of cadaveric donor grafts, an agonizing waiting period begins after the patient has been accepted as a transplant candidate. The family returns home and the wait begins for a suitable organ to be located. Once a match is made, the Transplant Center notifies the family and asks them to return to the center for surgery. The family is usually required to return to the Transplant Center at a moment's notice, so they may need to carry a pager and keep the Transplant Center aware of any changes in address or telephone number.

E. Pediatric Transplant Options

E.1. Living-donor transplantation

At University of Minnesota/Fairview-University Medical Center (F-UMC), we encourage living-donor transplantation. This approach is based on data showing that the outcomes of transplantation with living donors are better than those with cadaveric donors.[11] Approximately 70% to 75% of our grafts in children are from living donors. Living-donor transplantation may offer improved results due to better histocompatibility matching, decreased cold ischemic time, and the ability to schedule the transplant surgery for a period when the child's nutritional status is good.

We provide the potential donor with information pertaining to the risks of the procedure. We minimize stress and coercion on the part of family members. Approximately 30% of our patients have identified living donors by the time they reach end-stage kidney disease and are able to undergo preemptive kidney transplantation without a period of dialysis.

E.2. Cadaveric kidney waiting list

Patients without potential living donors go onto a waiting list for cadaveric kidney transplantation. While the transplant candidate is on this list, routine follow-up is essential to assess the course of the disease, adjust his or her medical status, if necessary, and address any new medical problems. It is very important for referring physicians and medical facilities to notify the Transplant Center if the candidate's condition significantly deteriorates, if secondary complications or new medical problems develop, or if hospitalization is required.

BLANCHE M. CHAVERS, MD, AND MARIE COOK, RN, CPNP, MPH, CCTC

References

1. Chavers BM, Matas AJ, Gillingham KJ, Schmidt WJ, Najarian JS. Pediatric renal transplantation at the University of Minnesota: the cyclosporine years. *Clin Transpl.* 1994:203-212.

2. Humar A, Nevins TE, Remucal M, Cook ME, Matas AJ, Najarian JS. Kidney transplantation in children younger than 1 year using cyclosporine immunosuppression. *Ann Surg.* 1998;228:421-428.

3. Papalois VE, Najarian JS. Pediatric kidney transplantation: historic hallmarks and a personal perspective. *Pediatr Transplant.* 2001;5:239-45.

4. U.S. Renal Data System. *USRDS 2000 Annual Data Report.* Bethesda, MD: The National Institutes of Health, National Institute of Diabetes and Digestive and Kidney Diseases; 2000.

5. Davis IB, Bunchman TE, Grimm PC, Benfield MR, Briscoe DM, Harmon WE, Alexander SR, Avner ED. Pediatric renal transplantation: Indications and special considerations. *Pediatr Transplant.* 1998;2:117-129.

6. Rotundo A, Nevins TE, Lipton M, Lockman LA, Mauer SM, Michael AF. Progressive encephalopathy in children with chronic renal insufficiency in infancy. *Kidney Int.* 1982;21:486-91.

7. Salvatierra O, Jr., Tanney D, Mak R, Alfrey E, Lemley K, Mackie F, So S, Hammer GB, Krane EJ, Conley SB. Pediatric renal transplantation and its challenges. *Transplantation Reviews.* 1997;11:51-69.

8. Khan K, Schwarzenberg SJ, Sharp HL, Matas AJ, Chavers BM. Morbidity from congenital hepatic fibrosis after renal transplantation for autosomal recessive polycystic kidney disease. *Am J Transplant.* 2002;2:360-365.

9. Matas AJ, Chavers BM, Nevins TE, Mauer SM, Kashtan CE, Cook M, Najarian JS. Recipient evaluation, preparation and care in pediatric transplantation: the University of Minnesota protocols. *Kidney Int.* 1996;49(suppl 53):S99-S102.

10. Miller RB, Burke BA, Schmidt WJ, Gillingham KJ, Matas AJ, Mauer M, Kashtan CE. Recurrence of haemolytic-uraemic syndrome in renal transplants: a single-center report. *Nephrol Dial Transplant.* 1997;12:1425-30.

11. Vats A, Gillingham K, Matas A, Chavers B. Improved late graft survival and half-lives in pediatric kidney transplantation: a single center experience. *Am J Transplant.* 2002;2(10):939-945.

Table 1. Current Immunosuppression at the University of Minnesota/Fairview-University Medical Center (F-UMC)

Drug	Dosage
Thymoglobulin	1.25-1.5 mg/kg intraoperatively 1.25-1.5 mg/kg on postoperative days 1-4
Prednisone	500 mg Solu-Medrol intraoperatively 1 mg/kg on postoperative day 1 0.5 mg/kg on postoperative days 2 and 3 0.25 mg/kg on postoperative days 4 and 5
Cyclosporine	4 mg/kg, BID, adjusted to achieve blood levels of 150-200 ng/mL for the first 3 months
CellCept	1 gm BID

Table 2. Usual Side Effects and Drug Interactions of Commonly Used Immunosuppressive Medications

	CsA/Tacrolimus	Azathioprine	Mycophenolate Mofetil
Common side effects	hypertension, nephrotoxicity, hirsutism (CsA), neurotoxicity, osteoporosis, hyperglycemia (tacrolimus), hepatotoxicity (unusual)	leukopenia, anemia, thrombocytopenia, GI upset, pancreatitis (unusual), hepatotoxicity (unusual)	leukopenia, thrombocytopenia, GI upset
Other medications that increase blood levels	azithromycin, clarithromycin, diltiazem, doxycycline, erythromycin, fluconazole, itraconazole, ketoconazole, nicardipine, verapamil, H_2 blockers	allopurinol	tacrolimus
Other medications that decrease blood levels	carbamazepine, isoniazid, octreotide, phenobarbital, phenytoin, rifampin, St. John's wort		cholestyramine, antacids (aluminum-, calcium-, and magnesium-based)
Other medications that potentiate toxicities	*nephrotoxicity:* acyclovir, aminoglycosides, amphotericin B, ACE inhibitors, colchicine, erythromycin, ganciclovir, H_2 blockers, NSAIDs, ciprofloxacin	*bone-marrow suppression:* allopurinol, sulfonamides, ganciclovir, cyclophosphamide, methotrexate	

ACE inhibitors = angiotensin-converting enzyme inhibitors
CsA = cyclosporine
GI = gastrointestinal
NSAIDs = nonsteroidal anti-inflammatory drugs

Table 2. Usual Side Effects and Drug Interactions of Commonly Used Immunosuppressive Medications (continued)

	PREDNISONE	SIROLIMUS (RAPAMYCIN)
Common side effects	weight gain, hyperglycemia, osteoporosis, cataracts, myopathy	anemia, thrombocytopenia, leukopenia, hypertension, peripheral edema, mouth sores, hypercholesterolemia, hypertriglyceridemia, hypokalemia, headache
Other medications that increase blood levels		azithromycin, clarithromycin, fluconazole, ketoconazole, itraconazole, erythromycin, diltiazem, nicardipine, verapamil, cimetidine, CsA
Other medications that decrease blood levels		carbamazepine, isoniazid, phenobarbital, phenytoin, rifampin, rifapentine, rifabutin
Other medications that potentiate toxicities		

CsA = cyclosporine

Table 3. Cyclosporine (CsA) and Tacrolimus Drug Interactions

DRUG	PROPOSED MECHANISM	POSSIBLE EFFECT	COMMENTS
Dietary Factors			
Grapefruit juice	Decreased metabolism	Increased blood concentration	Consistency in nature of foods with which CsA is taken
Dietary fat	Increased bioavailability	Increased blood concentration	Consistency in nature of foods with which CsA is taken
Enteral feeding	Decreased bioavailability by inducing diarrhea	Decreased blood concentration	Monitor stool output, drug levels
St. John's wort	Increased metabolism	Decreased blood concentration	Monitor levels; may need to increase dose
Sex Hormones			
Danazol	Decreased metabolism	Increased blood concentration with increased nephrotoxicity and hepatotoxicity	Avoid, if possible. Immediately decrease dose
Methyltestosterone	Decreased metabolism	Increased blood concentration with increased nephrotoxicity and hepatotoxicity	Monitor concentration and for signs/symptoms of toxicity
Oral contraceptives (levonorgestrel and ethinyl estradiol)	Decreased metabolism	Increased blood concentration with increased hepatotoxicity	LFTs and bilirubin should be monitored
Norethandrolone	Decreased metabolism	Increased hepatotoxicity	LFTs and bilirubin should be monitored

CsA = cyclosporine   LFTs = liver function tests

Table 3. Cyclosporine (CsA) and Tacrolimus Drug Interactions (continued)

Drug	Proposed Mechanism	Possible Effect	Comments
Tamoxifen	Decreased metabolism (in vitro)	Increased blood concentration	Monitor concentration and signs/symptoms of toxicity
Anticonvulsant Agents			
Carbamazepine	Increased metabolism	Decreased blood concentration with associated rejection of transplanted organ	Alternative: valproate or immediate increase in dose; monitor concentrations. At offset, monitor concentrations
Phenobarbital	Increased metabolism	Decreased blood concentration with associated rejection of transplanted organ	Alternative: valproate
Phenytoin	Increased metabolism	Decreased blood concentration with associated rejection of transplanted organ. Also, increased gingival hyperplasia	Alternative: valproate. Increase dose
Primidone	Increased metabolism	Decreased blood concentration	
Gastrointestinal Agents			
Antacids	Decreased absorption	Decreased blood concentration	Separate doses. Alternatives: ranitidine, famotidine, lansoprazole, and omeprazole
Bile acids	Increased bioavailability (Sandimmune)	Increased blood concentration	Monitor concentrations and for signs/symptoms of toxicity
Cimetidine	Decreased metabolism	Increased blood concentration and increased creatinine (controversial)	Alternatives: ranitidine, famotidine, lansoprazole, and omeprazole

Table 3. Cyclosporine (CsA) and Tacrolimus Drug Interactions (continued)

Drug	Proposed Mechanism	Possible Effect	Comments
Metoclopramide	Increased bioavailability	Increased blood concentration	Clinical significance controversial
Octreotide	Decreased bioavailability	Decreased blood concentration	Clinical significance controversial
Omeprazole	Decreased metabolism (*in vitro*)	Increased blood concentration	Clinical significance controversial
Cardiovascular Agents			
Amiodarone	Decreased metabolism	Increased blood concentration	Monitor concentration and for signs/symptoms of toxicity
ACE inhibitors	Altered renal vascular tone	Increased nephrotoxicity (controversial) except enalapril may have protective renal effects	When an acceptable alternative is not available, monitor closely for signs of nephrotoxicity
Diltiazem	Decreased metabolism	Increased blood concentration	Decrease dose by 50%–80%. Alternatives: isradipine, felodipine, prazosin
Disopyramide	Unknown	Increased creatinine	Monitor closely for signs of nephrotoxicity
Furosemide	Sodium depletion	Increased nephrotoxicity (animals)	Monitor closely for signs of nephrotoxicity

ACE inhibitors = angiotensin-converting enzyme inhibitors

Table 3. Cyclosporine (CsA) and Tacrolimus Drug Interactions (continued)

Drug	Proposed Mechanism	Possible Effect	Comments
HMG-CoA reductase inhibitors (lovastatin, simvastatin, atorvastatin, pravastatin, cerivastatin)	Decreased metabolism of HMG-CoA reductase inhibitor, decreased clearance	Myositis and elevation in CK	Monitor CK, symptoms of myositis and/or myalgias; use lowest effective daily dose. Pravastatin may have lesser effect
Mannitol	Unknown	Increased nephrotoxicity (animals)	Monitor closely for signs of nephrotoxicity
Nicardipine	Decreased metabolism	Increased blood concentration	Monitor concentration. Alternatives: diltiazem, amlodipine, isradipine, prazosin
Nifedipine	Decreased metabolism (tacrolimus) Unknown	Increased blood concentration gingival hyperplasia	Monitor concentration. Alternatives: amlodipine, isradipine, prazosin
Prazosin	Renal protective effects	Reduced nephrotoxicity	
Propranolol	Unknown	Antagonistic immunosuppressive effects (animals)	
Spironolactone	Unknown	Renal protective effects	

CK = creatine kinase

Table 3. Cyclosporine (CsA) and Tacrolimus Drug Interactions (continued)

Drug	Proposed Mechanism	Possible Effect	Comments
Steroids			
Corticosterone	Decreased metabolism Unknown	Increased blood concentration Increased neurotoxicity with ketoconazole	Monitor levels frequently in patients receiving high doses of methylprednisolone (>250 mg/d). Monitor for signs/symptoms of nephrotoxicity/neurotoxicity
Dexamethasone	Decreased metabolism	Increased blood concentration	Clinical significance controversial
Prednisolone	Decreased metabolism Decreased prednisolone metabolism	Increased blood concentration Increased prednisolone concentration	Clinical significance controversial
Miscellaneous			
Alcohol (heavy intake)	Decreased metabolism	Increased blood concentration	
Astemizole	Decreased astemizole metabolism	Cardiac arrhythmias	Avoid combination
Atracurium	Unknown	Enhanced neuromuscular blockade	Monitor depth of neuromuscular blockade
Bromocriptine	Decreased metabolism	Increased blood concentration	
Cisplatin	Nephrotoxic agent	Increased nephrotoxicity	
Cyclosporine	Decreased metabolism (tacrolimus)	Increased blood concentration and increased nephrotoxicity	Avoid combination
Ergotamine	Decreased metabolism	Increased blood concentration	
Etoposide	Unknown	Increased cytotoxicity	

Table 3. Cyclosporine (CsA) and Tacrolimus Drug Interactions (continued)

Drug	Proposed Mechanism	Possible Effect	Comments
Fentanyl	Unknown	Increased analgesia	
Melphalan	Unknown	Increased nephrotoxicity	
Midazolam	Decreased metabolism	Increased blood concentration	
Tacrolimus	Decreased metabolism (CsA)	Increased blood concentration and increased nephrotoxicity	Avoid combination
Vecuronium	Unknown	Enhanced neuromuscular blockade	
Nonsteroidal and Other Anti-inflammatory Agents			
Colchicine	Unknown	Increased nephrotoxicity	
Diclofenac	Reduced prostaglandin production	Increased nephrotoxicity	
Indomethacin	Reduced prostaglandin production	Increased nephrotoxicity	
NSAIDs	Reduced prostaglandin production	Increased nephrotoxicity	Avoid combination
Sulindac	Unknown and reduced prostaglandin production	Increased blood concentration and increased nephrotoxicity	
Anti-infective Agents			
Acyclovir	Nephrotoxic agent	Increased nephrotoxicity, mostly with IV use	When an acceptable alternative is not available, monitor closely for signs of nephrotoxicity

CsA = cyclosporine   NSAIDS = nonsteroidal anti-inflammatory drugs   IV = intravenous

Table 3. Cyclosporine (CsA) and Tacrolimus Drug Interactions (continued)

Drug	Proposed Mechanism	Possible Effect	Comments
Aminoglycosides	Nephrotoxic agent	Increased nephrotoxicity	When an acceptable alternative is not available, monitor closely for signs of nephrotoxicity
Amphotericin B	Nephrotoxic agent Unknown	Increased nephrotoxicity Increased hepatotoxicity	When an acceptable alternative is not available, use sodium loading, liposomal amphotericin; monitor closely
Azithromycin, Clarithromycin	Decreased metabolism	Increased blood concentration with increased nephrotoxicity	Use alternative antibiotic, if possible
Ciprofloxacin	Nephrotoxic agent	Increased nephrotoxicity	Alternative: cephalosporins
Clotrimazole	Decreased metabolism	Increased blood concentration	
Co-trimoxazole (trimethoprim/ sulfamethoxazole)	Nephrotoxic agent and tubular effect on creatinine	Increased nephrotoxicity and increased serum creatinine with higher dosages	When an acceptable alternative is not available, monitor closely for signs of nephrotoxicity
Doxycycline	Unknown	Increased blood concentration	
Erythromycin	Decreased metabolism	Increased blood concentration	Decrease dose by 50%
Fluconazole	Decreased metabolism (dose dependent)	Increased blood concentration	Decrease dose by 50%, monitor levels
Ganciclovir	Nephrotoxic agent	Increased nephrotoxicity	
Imipenem	Decreased metabolism	Increased blood concentration and enhanced neurotoxicity	
Indinavir	Decreased metabolism	Increased blood concentration	Decrease dose by 50%, monitor levels

Table 3. Cyclosporine (CsA) and Tacrolimus Drug Interactions (continued)

DRUG	PROPOSED MECHANISM	POSSIBLE EFFECT	COMMENTS
Itraconazole	Decreased metabolism	Increased blood concentration	Immediately reduce dose by 50%; monitor levels frequently until new steady-state is reached. When itraconazole is stopped; monitor levels and increase dose accordingly
Ketoconazole	Decreased metabolism	Increased blood concentration with increased nephrotoxicity	Immediately reduce dose by 50%, with subsequent dose adjustments
Nafcillin	Increased metabolism	Decreased blood concentration	Alternative: cephalosporins
Norfloxacin	Decreased metabolism (conflicting data)	Increased blood concentration	
Rifampin	Increased metabolism	Decreased blood concentration with associated rejection of transplanted organ	Monitor concentration and adjust dose accordingly. Dose increase, as much as 2-3 times, may be necessary.
Ritonavir	Decreased metabolism	Increased blood concentration	Decrease dose by 50%, monitor levels
Saquinavir	Decreased metabolism	Increased blood concentration	Decrease dose by 50%, monitor levels
Ticarcillin	Unknown	Increased blood concentration	
Psychotropic Agents			
Fluvoxamine	Decreased metabolism	Increased blood concentration	Alternatives: paroxetine, venlafaxine, citalopram
Nefazadone	Decreased metabolism	Increased blood concentration	Alternatives: paroxetine, venlafaxine, citalopram

Table 4. Azathioprine (AZA) Drug Interactions

Drug	Proposed Mechanism	Possible Effect	Comments
Allopurinol	Decreased metabolism	Severe leukopenia. Recovery of WBC may take up to 4-8 weeks	Avoid if preferable. AZA dose reduction of 75%-80% needed to avoid severe leukopenia
Cyclophosphamide	Potentiation of bone-marrow suppressive effects	Leukopenia, anemia, thrombocytopenia	Monitor CBC
Ganciclovir	Potentiation of bone-marrow suppressive effects	Leukopenia, anemia, thrombocytopenia	Monitor CBC
Methotrexate	Potentiation of bone-marrow suppressive effects	Leukopenia, anemia, thrombocytopenia	Monitor CBC
Pancuronium	Unknown	Reduced neuromuscular blockade	May require dose increase of pancuronium
Succinylcholine	Unknown	Enhanced neuromuscular blockade	Dose reduction of succinylcholine may be needed
Sulfonamides	Potentiation of bone-marrow suppressive effects	Leukopenia, anemia, thrombocytopenia	Monitor CBC
Warfarin	Increased warfarin metabolism	Increased dose requirements of warfarin have been reported in 6-mercaptopurine-treated patients	

AZA = azathioprine   CBC = complete blood count   WBC = white blood cells

Table 5. Mycophenolate Mofetil (MMF) Drug Interactions

Drug	Proposed Mechanism	Possible Effect	Comments
Acyclovir	Decreased metabolism	Increased AUC of MPA glucuronide. Increase in acyclovir concentration	Decrease acyclovir dose by 20% when given with MMF; clinical significance controversial
Antacids	Decreased bioavailability	Decreased AUC of MPA by 33%	Give antacid 2 hours after MMF
Cholestyramine	Decreased bioavailability	Decreased AUC of MPA by 40%	Do not administer cholestyramine with MMF
Phenytoin	Protein-binding displacement of phenytoin	Displaces phenytoin from binding sites	Monitor total and free phenytoin concentrations
Salicylates	Protein-binding displacement	Displaces MPA from albumin binding sites	Monitor salicylate concentrations and for signs of salicylate toxicity
Tacrolimus	Decreased metabolism	Increased MMF trough concentration by decreased glucuronidation or increased glucuronidase activity	Monitor CBC
Theophylline	Protein-binding displacement of theophylline	Displaces theophylline from binding sites	Monitor theophylline concentrations and for signs of toxicity

AUC = area under the curve
CBC = complete blood count
MMF = mycophenolate mofetil
MPA = mycophenolic acid

Table 6. Sirolimus (Rapamycin) Drug Interactions*

DRUG	PROPOSED MECHANISM	POSSIBLE EFFECT	COMMENTS
Sex Hormones			
Danazol	Inhibition of sirolimus metabolism	Increased sirolimus levels	Monitor levels closely; use these drugs together with caution
Anticonvulsant Agents			
Carbamazepine	Induction of sirolimus metabolism	Decreased sirolimus levels	Monitor levels closely; use these drugs together with caution
Phenobarbital	Induction of sirolimus metabolism	Decreased sirolimus levels	Monitor levels closely; use these drugs together with caution
Phenytoin	Induction of sirolimus metabolism	Decreased sirolimus levels	Monitor levels closely; use these drugs together with caution
Gastrointestinal Agents			
Cimetidine	Inhibition of sirolimus metabolism	Increased sirolimus levels	Monitor levels closely; use these drugs together with caution

*Drugs known to affect cyclosporine (CsA) or tacrolimus metabolism will probably also affect the metabolism of sirolimus. If medications known to affect CsA or tacrolimus metabolism are given to a patient on sirolimus, a dosage adjustment may be necessary.

Table 6. Sirolimus (Rapamycin) Drug Interactions* (continued)

DRUG	PROPOSED MECHANISM	POSSIBLE EFFECT	COMMENTS
Cardiovascular Agents			
Diltiazem	Inhibition of sirolimus metabolism	Increased sirolimus levels	Monitor levels closely; use these drugs together with caution
Nicardipine	Inhibition of sirolimus metabolism	Increased sirolimus levels	Monitor levels closely; use these drugs together with caution
Verapamil	Inhibition of sirolimus metabolism	Increased sirolimus levels	Monitor levels closely; use these drugs together with caution
Miscellaneous Agents			
Bromocriptine	Inhibition of sirolimus metabolism	Increased sirolimus levels	Monitor levels closely; use these drugs together with caution
Cyclosporine	Inhibition of sirolimus metabolism	Increased sirolimus levels	Monitor levels closely; use these drugs together with caution; administer sirolimus 4 hours after CsA dose if not routinely monitoring sirolimus levels
Anti-infective Agents			
Azithromycin	Inhibition of sirolimus metabolism	Increased sirolimus levels	Monitor levels closely; use these drugs together with caution

*Drugs known to affect cyclosporine (CsA) or tacrolimus metabolism will probably also affect the metabolism of sirolimus. If medications known to affect CsA or tacrolimus metabolism are given to a patient on sirolimus, a dosage adjustment may be necessary.

Table 6. Sirolimus (Rapamycin) Drug Interactions* (continued)

DRUG	PROPOSED MECHANISM	POSSIBLE EFFECT	COMMENTS
Clarithromycin	Inhibition of sirolimus metabolism	Increased sirolimus levels	Monitor levels closely; use these drugs together with caution
Erythromycin	Inhibition of sirolimus metabolism	Increased sirolimus levels	Monitor levels closely; use these drugs together with caution
Fluconazole	Inhibition of sirolimus metabolism	Increased sirolimus levels	Monitor levels closely; use these drugs together with caution
Indinavir	Inhibition of sirolimus metabolism	Increased sirolimus levels	Monitor levels closely; use these drugs together with caution
Itraconazole	Inhibition of sirolimus metabolism	Increased sirolimus levels	Monitor levels closely; use these drugs together with caution
Ketoconazole	Inhibition of sirolimus metabolism	Major increase in sirolimus levels	Not recommended to use these drugs together
Rifabutin	Induction of sirolimus metabolism	Decreased sirolimus levels	Monitor levels closely; use these drugs together with caution
Rifampin	Induction of sirolimus metabolism	Decreased sirolimus levels	Monitor levels closely; use these drugs together with caution

*Drugs known to affect cyclosporine (CsA) or tacrolimus metabolism will probably also affect the metabolism of sirolimus. If medications known to affect CsA or tacrolimus metabolism are given to a patient on sirolimus, a dosage adjustment may be necessary.

Table 6. Sirolimus (Rapamycin) Drug Interactions* (continued)

DRUG	PROPOSED MECHANISM	POSSIBLE EFFECT	COMMENTS
Rifapentine	Induction of sirolimus metabolism	Decreased sirolimus levels	Monitor levels closely; use these drugs together with caution
Ritonavir	Inhibition of sirolimus metabolism	Increased sirolimus levels	Monitor levels closely; use these drugs together with caution
Troleandromycin	Inhibition of sirolimus metabolism	Increased sirolimus levels	Monitor levels closely; use these drugs together with caution

*Drugs known to affect cyclosporine (CsA) or tacrolimus metabolism will probably also affect the metabolism of sirolimus. If medications known to affect CsA or tacrolimus metabolism are given to a patient on sirolimus, a dosage adjustment may be necessary.

Table 7. Prednisone Drug Interactions

DRUG	PROPOSED MECHANISM	POSSIBLE EFFECT	COMMENTS
Oral contraceptives	Increased metabolism	Increased potential for adverse steroid effects	
Phenytoin	Increased metabolism	Reduced immunosuppressive actions with reduced graft-survival rates	Give dose in two divided dosages
Phenobarbital	Increased metabolism	Reduced immunosuppressive actions with reduced graft-survival rates	
Rifampin	Increased metabolism and reduced bioavailability of prednisolone	Reduced immunosuppressive actions with reduced graft-survival rates	

Table 8. Use of Immunosuppressive Medications in Dialysis Patients

EFFECT OF DIALYSIS	MEDICATION
Removed by dialysis (administer after dialysis)	Azathioprine.
Not removed by dialysis	Cyclosporine, tacrolimus, sirolimus (rapamycin), mycophenolate mofetil, prednisone, polyclonal antilymphocyte globulins (Atgam, Thymoglobulin) OKT3, basiliximab, daclizumab

Table 9. Evaluation of the Pediatric Renal Transplant Recipient at the University of Minnesota/Fairview-University Medical Center

1. Perform a detailed history and physical examination.

2. Document growth data.

3. Conduct tests of renal, hepatic, and coagulation function.

4. Screen for cytomegalovirus (CMV), Epstein-Barr virus (EBV), herpes virus, human immunodeficiency virus (HIV), hepatitis A, B, and C, varicella-zoster virus, and measles/mumps/rubella antibody.

5. Evaluate and treat for renal osteodystrophy.

6. Obtain ABO, tissue typing, and antileukocyte antibody screening.

7. Obtain consults from appropriate services such as social service, pediatric neurology, dentistry, pediatric psychology, nutrition, and pediatric urology.

8. Obtain urine cultures; examine for evidence of peritoneal catheter exit site and/or tunnel infection.

9. Obtain chest radiograph and bone age films.

10. Obtain an electrocardiogram and a cardiac echocardiogram, when indicated.

11. Obtain voiding cystourethrogram.

12. Obtain Pap smear in adolescent girls older than 15 years of age.

13. Document immunization history and administer childhood immunizations, when indicated.

14. Place a TB skin test with controls for mumps and *Candida*.

15. Administer hepatitis B, pneumococcal, and varicella vaccinations, when indicated.

16. Evaluate for hypertension and treat when indicated.

17. Direct patient to attend pretransplant class and clinic for education regarding transplantation procedures, transplant medications, and posttransplant monitoring.

18. Complete pretransplant checklist.

Glossary of Abbreviations and Acronyms

ACE: angiotensin-converting enzyme

ACR: albumin-to-creatinine ratio

ADA: American Diabetes Association

Alb: serum albumin concentration

ALT: alanine aminotransferase

AR: acute rejection

ARPKD: autosomal recessive polycystic kidney disease

AST: aspartate aminotransferase

ATN: acute tubular necrosis

AUC: area under curve

AUC_{12}: area under concentration-time curve over 12 hours

AZA: azathioprine

BID: twice daily

BMI: body mass index

BP: blood pressure

BUN: blood urea nitrogen

CAD: coronary artery disease

CBC: complete blood count

C_{CR}: creatinine clearance

CD4 cells: T-helper cells

CK: creatine kinase

CMV: cytomegalovirus

CNS: central nervous system

Cr: creatinine

CR: chronic rejection

CsA: cyclosporine

CT: computed tomography

CVD: cardiovascular disease

CVP: central venous pressure

D5W: 5% dextrose

DGF: delayed graft function

DMS: diffuse mesangial sclerosis

DNA: deoxyribonucleic acid

DVT: deep venous thrombosis

EBV: Epstein-Barr virus

ECG: electrocardiogram

ESRD: end-stage renal disease

FDA: Food and Drug Administration

FK: FK506 (tacrolimus)

FKBP12: FK-binding protein 12

FSGS: focal segmental glomerulosclerosis

F-UMC: Fairview-University Medical Center

GFR: glomerular filtration rate

GGT: gamma-glutamyltransferase

GI: gastrointestinal

GN: glomerulonephritis

HAMA: human anti-mouse antibody

Hb_sAg: hepatitis B surface antigen

HBV: hepatitis B virus

HCV: hepatitis C virus

Hgb: hemoglobin

HIV: human immunodeficiency virus

HLA: human leukocyte antigen

HMG-CoA: 3-hydroxy-3-methylglutaryl-co-enzyme A

HPLC: high-performance liquid chromatography

HUS: hemolytic uremic syndrome

IGF: immediate graft function

IL-2: interleukin-2

INH: isoniazid

INR: international normalized ratio

IRB: institutional review board

IV: intravenous(ly)

LDKT: living-donor kidney transplant(ation)

LDL: low-density lipoprotein

LFTs: liver function tests

MDRD: Modification of Diet in Renal Disease

MIS: minimally invasive surgery

MMF: mycophenolate mofetil

MPA: mycophenolic acid

MRI: magnetic resonance imaging

mTOR: mammalian target of rapamycin

NPO: nothing by os (nothing by mouth)

NS: normal saline

NSAIDs: nonsteroidal anti-inflammatory drugs

OKT3: muromonab-CD3

PA: posteroanterior
PCP: *Pneumocystis carinii* pneumonia
P$_{CR}$: serum creatinine concentration
PE: pulmonary embolism
PFA: patient financial advocate
PFR: patient financial representative
PO: per os (orally)
POD: postoperative day
PPD: purified protein derivative
PRA: panel reactive antibody
PSA: prostate-specific antigen
PT: prothrombin time
PTD: percutaneous transluminal dilation
PTLD: posttransplant lymphoproliferative
   disease
PTT: partial thromboplastin time
PUD: peptic ulcer disease
PVD: peripheral vascular disease
RAT: renal artery thrombosis
RIA: radioimmunoassay
RPR: rapid plasma reagin
RRT: renal replacement therapy
SGF: slow graft function
SUN: serum urea nitrogen concentration
TIA: transient ischemic attack
TMP/SMX: trimethoprim-
   sulfamethoxazole
TNF: tumor necrosis factor
UNOS: United Network for Organ Sharing
VCUG: voiding cystourethrogram
WBC: white blood cell(s)

Index

6-antigen matched kidney, 5

abscess, 33, 36, 104
absorption, 33, 38, 43, 51, 77, 98, 116
absorption profiling, 74, 77; CSA, 89; sirolimus, 51; tacrolimus, 43, 77
abstinence, 79, 99
accelerated rejection, 34
accommodations, 12
acetaminophen, 58, 62
acne, 54
acute liver (hepatic) failure, 6, 34-35, 38, 40, 46, 60, 65, 73, 78, 83-84, 88, 90, 95-100, 102-103, 109, 111, 131
acute rejection (AR), 28-31, 34, 56, 59, 68, 70-71, 73, 76-77, 87, 89-90, 132
acute tubular necrosis (ATN), 25-27, 35, 132
alanine aminotransferase (ALT), 40, 78, 132
albumin, 8, 38, 43, 46, 75-77, 92, 97, 102, 104, 124; excretion, 77; level, 83
albumin-to-creatinine ratio, 75, 77, 132
alcohol abuse, 15, 119
alkaline phosphatase, 75, 78
allergic reaction, 46, 61
alopecia, 44
Alport's syndrome, 96
amylase, 8
anaphylaxis, 57, 63, 65-66
anastomoses, 24-25, 33; end-to-end, 24; end-to-side, 24
anemia, 46-47, 78, 97-98, 109, 113-114, 123
angina, 60
angiography, 7
angiotensin-converting enzyme (ACE) inhibitor, 78, 81, 113,

117, 132
antacids, 36, 50, 55, 113, 116, 124
antihypertensive agents, 80-81, 100
anti-T cell modulating agents, 35, 56
anti-thymocyte globulin-rabbit (Thymoglobulin), 34, 56-59, 63, 68, 71, 112, 130
antibiotics, 33, 104, 121
antibody, 8, 29, 56, 58, 60-61, 63, 65, 86-87, 104, 108, 131-133; cytotoxic, 48, 56; monoclonal, 59, 63-65; polyclonal, 56, 70, 72
antigen, 8-9, 16, 56, 59, 85, 104, 132-133
antilymphocyte agents, 30, 34, 130
anuria, 27
aphthous ulcers, 52
area under curve (AUC), 39, 75, 124, 132
area under drug concentration-time curve over 12 hours (AUC₁₂), 77-78, 132
arrhythmias, 119
aspartate aminotransferase (AST), 40, 78, 132
aspirin, 79, 90-91
atovaquone, 87
atresia, 99
autosomal recessive polycystic kidney disease (ARPKD), 103, 111, 132
azathioprine (AZA), 30, 45-48, 67, 70, 113, 123, 130, 132; Imuran, 37, 45
azithromycin, 42, 45, 113-114, 121, 126

bacterial infections, 61
basiliximab (Simulect), 64-66, 69, 130

beta-blockers, 81
bilateral nephrectomy, 100-101, 103
bile, 38, 116
bilirubin, 8, 40, 75, 78, 104, 115; direct, 75
bioavailability, 38, 43, 50-51, 115-117, 124, 129
biopsy, 6, 23, 29, 34, 103, 109
biphosphonate therapy, 55
bladder, 33, 84, 102-103; competency, 101; distension, 101; dysfunction, 101; irrigation, 33; storage capacity, 101
bleeding, 26-27, 31, 33, 36, 103
blindness, 61
blood pressure, 26, 54, 75, 80, 104, 132; diastolic, 80; high, 15; monitoring, 62; systolic, 25
blood screening, ABO blood group typing, 131; antileukocyte antibody screening, 104, 131; cross-matching, 8, 16, 34, 58, 99, 108; HLA typing, 104
blood, drug concentration monitoring, 38, 44, 99, 115-122
blood clots, 32-33, 104, 121
blood sugar, 35, 54, 75, 81, 92, 97
blood urea nitrogen (BUN), 8, 16, 28, 75, 99, 104, 132
body mass index (BMI), 22-23, 132
bone, 81-82, 91, 97-98, 103, 113, 123; age, 105, 131; fractures, 98; mineral density, 81; disease, 81, 97-98
bowel dysfunction, 21

breast cancer, 83, 85, 92
breast examination, 8, 16, 85
bronchoscopy, 35
burning, 40

cadaver, 108
cadaveric kidney transplant, 5, 7, 9, 15, 28-29, 70, 84, 100, 108-110
calcineurin, 37
calcineurin inhibitor, 30, 80, 82; CSA (Neoral, Gengraf, Eon), 30, 37; tacrolimus (Prograf), 30
calcium, 27, 55, 75, 82, 91, 97-99, 104, 113; level, 81-82, 98; supplementation, 102
calcium channel blockers, 27
cancer, 6, 15-16, 73, 83, 85, 92-93, 99; contraindication, 99. *See also* specific cancers.
cancer screening tests, 85; colonoscopy, 85; flexible sigmoidoscopy, 85; mammogram, 8, 16, 85; Pap, 8, 16, 85, 92, 105, 131; PSA, 8, 16, 85, 133
Candida infections, 9, 105, 131; esophagitis, 87; oral thrush, 87
candidiasis, 54, 87
capsules, 41-42, 44, 49
carbon dioxide, 22, 75
cardiac arrest, 28
cardiac complications, 13, 34; hypertension, 15, 27, 31, 34-35, 40, 44, 54, 61, 80, 89, 96, 100, 103, 113-114, 131; myocardial infarction, 26, 34, 60, 79, 90-91; pericarditis, 34
cardiac evaluation, 6
cardiac failure, 35, 65

Index

(MDRD), 5-6, 132
mood alterations, 54
mumps, 9, 104-105, 131
Muromonab-CD3 (OKT3), 34-35, 59-63, 68, 130, 132
muscle, 91; cramps, 54; wasting, 54; weakness, 54, 82, 98
mycophenolate mofetil (MMF), 30, 46-50, 52, 67, 78, 90, 113, 124, 130, 132; CellCept, 37, 47-48, 71-72, 112
mycophenolic acid (MPA), 48, 50, 67, 75, 78, 90, 124, 132
mycostatin troches, 87
myelosuppression, 46
myocardial infarction, 34, 60, 79, 90-91

National Kidney Foundation, 89; chronic kidney disease stages, 5; classification, 5; guidelines, 5
native nephrectomy, 100
nausea, 21, 46, 48, 52, 60, 96
nebulizer treatments, 62
Neoral, 37-39, 41-42, 67, 71, 89
nephrectomy, bilateral, 100-101, 103; laparoscopic, 20-23; native, 80, 100; open donor, 20-22
nephrocalcinosis, 102
nephromegaly, 103
nephrotic syndromes, 94, 100-101; congenital nephrotic syndrome, 96, 101; diffuse mesangial sclerosis, 101, 132; focal segmental glomerulosclerosis, 6, 96, 101, 109, 132
nephrotoxicity, 30, 34, 38-40, 44, 52, 89, 113, 115, 117-122
nephroureterectomy, 100

neuraminidase inhibitor, 86
neurotoxicity, 40, 44, 113, 119, 121
noncompliance (with medical management), 9-10, 34, 73, 99
normal saline (NS), 41, 47, 57, 59, 64, 66, 132
numbness, 1-3, 6, 11, 24, 40, 56, 61, 70, 75-77, 80, 82, 84, 94, 109
nutrition, 83, 97, 131; adequacy of, 97; supplementation, 97, 102

obesity, 9, 22-23, 81, 83
OKT3, 34-35, 59-63, 68, 130, 132
oliguria, 34
open donor nephrectomy, 20-22
operative procedure, 23, 30
oral administration, 38, 49, 68
oral dose, 41, 44, 47, 49, 68, 86
oral suspension, 41
organ donation, 3, 7, 15, 18
organ procurement, 3
osteoporosis, 54-55, 81, 113-114
outpatient pharmacy, 11
outpatients, 11, 74, 88, 103
oxalate, 102
oxalosis, 5-6, 94, 96, 102
oxygen therapy, 26, 62

pancreas-kidney transplantation, 23-24
pancreatitis, 46, 48, 113
panel reactive antibody (PRA), 8, 29, 133
Pap smear, 8, 16, 85, 105, 131
parathyroidectomy, 82, 91
partial thromboplastin time (PTT), 8, 16, 133

patient/family education, 74, 103, 107
patient financial representative (PFR), 11, 133
patient history, 103-104
pediatric kidney transplantation, 1-3, 5-6, 24-25, 37, 47, 66, 94-111, 131; contraindications, 99-100, 106; indications, 96, 100, 111; options, 110; team, 94
pelvic examination, 8, 85
pentamidine, 87
peptic ulcer disease (PUD), 36, 133
percutaneous aspiration, 33
percutaneous drainage, 33
percutaneous kidney biopsy, 23
percutaneous nephrostomy, 32
percutaneous transluminal dilation (PTD), 32, 133
pericardiocentesis, 35
pericarditis, 34
perioperative, 34-35
peripheral vascular disease (PVD), 8, 31, 79, 133
peritoneal, 12, 102, 104-105, 131; cavity, 33; window, 33
peritonitis, 12, 104
pharmacist, 11-12, 107
pharmacy, 11-12, 64, 66
phlebitis, 57
phosphate, 91, 97; binders, 97; levels, 27, 98
phosphorus, 8, 75, 82
physical examination, 1, 6-7, 9-13, 15-19, 21-22, 34, 37, 51, 68, 74, 94, 96, 99-100, 102-104, 107, 109-110, 112, 131-132

platelets, 16, 52, 75, 78, 104
pneumococcal infection, 9, 86, 131
Pneumocystis carinii pneumonia (PCP), 61, 87, 132
pneumonia, 35, 61, 87, 132
Pneumovax, 9
polycystic kidney disease, 96, 103, 111, 132
polyuria, 27
portal hypertension, 103
portal shunting, 103
posterior urethral valves, 101-102
posttransplant care, 1, 10, 27-30, 32-35, 73-74, 76-93; frequency, 75; immediate, 26, 36; long-term, 31, 73. *See also* posttransplant medical complications; posttransplant surgical complications.
posttransplant follow-up, 10, 73-93
posttransplant lymphoproliferative disorder (PTLD), 57, 61, 63, 85, 133
posttransplant malignancies, 73, 83-85, 92
posttransplant medical complications, 1, 3, 7, 10-12, 25-36, 39, 49, 52, 54-55, 57, 61, 63, 67-68, 70-94, 99, 101-102, 104, 107-108, 131, 133
posttransplant surgical complications, 26, 30-31, 33-36, 73-75, 78, 83, 94, 105, 108
potassium, 27, 35, 75, 81-82, 99
prednisolone, 37, 53, 55, 119, 129
prednisone, 30, 37, 53-